Balancing Hormones, Easing Symptoms: A 28-Day Plan to Relieve Estrogen Dominance

Balancing Hormones, Easing Symptoms: A 28-Day Plan to Relieve Estrogen Dominance

Copyright © 2024 by **Omolola Habib (NMD)**

All rights reserved. No part of this publication may be reproduced, distributed, or transmitted in any form or by any means, including photocopying, recording, or other electronic or mechanical methods, without the prior written permission of the publisher, except in the case of brief quotations embodied in critical reviews and certain other noncommercial uses permitted by copyright law.

Table of Content

INTRODUCTION   4

CHAPTER 1: UNDERSTANDING THE ESTROGEN BALANCE   10

CHAPTER 2: THE 28-DAY PLAN TO RELIEVE ESTROGEN DOMINANCE   17

CHAPTER 3: REDUCING EXPOSURE TO ESTROGEN-LIKE COMPOUNDS   78

CHAPTER 4: SUPPORTING ESTROGEN METABOLISM AND ELIMINATION   90

CHAPTER 5: THE CRITICAL ROLES OF NUTRITION AND DIET   99

CHAPTER 6: BEYOND THE 28 DAYS - STRATEGIES FOR HORMONAL BALANCE   111

CONCLUSION   122

ABOUT THE AUTHOR   126

Introduction

What is Estrogen Dominance and Its Impact

Estrogen dominance occurs when there is an imbalance between estrogen and progesterone levels in the body, with higher estrogen exerting dominant effects. While estrogen is an important hormone for both women and men, too much of it can cause an array of unpleasant symptoms and increase future health risks.

Some key impacts of high estrogen relative to progesterone include:

- Weight gain and fluid retention
- Fibrocystic breasts and breast tenderness
- Mood swings, irritability and anxiety
- Irregular periods, heavy bleeding and clotting
- Fatigue and low motivation
- Reduced sex drive
- Hair loss and thinning hair
- Cold hands and feet
- Foggy thinking and memory lapses
- Headaches and migraines
- Sleep disturbances

- Yeast infections and urinary tract infections

In the long run, sustained estrogen dominance has been associated with higher incidence of female cancers like breast, ovarian and uterine cancers. It can also increase your risk of blood clots or cardiovascular issues in both men and women.

Balancing estrogen levels also plays a big role in fertility and getting pregnant. Excess estrogen can obstruct regular ovulation, egg quality and implantation for trying to conceive women.

As you can see, both the immediate uncomfortable symptoms as well as long term disease risks make this hormone imbalance an important one to address.

Symptoms of Estrogen Dominance

Some key signs and symptoms to know if you may be experiencing estrogen dominance:

1. Irregular, Heavy or Painful Periods

Excess estrogen exposure works on the uterine lining, causing a thicker than normal lining which eventual sheds in the form of heavy, prolonged and painful periods with dark colored blood clots.

Similarly, periods may become further apart as estrogen disrupts the feedback loop that controls regular ovulation each month.

2. Fibrocystic Breasts and Breast Tenderness

Swollen or tender breasts before your period are driven by the estrogen-progesterone imbalance. Excess estrogen fuels fluid retention and cyst formation, causing painful and dense breast tissue.

Beyond PMS symptoms, this also increases lifetime risk of fibroids or breast cancer.

3. Weight Gain and Fluid Retention

Gaining weight in the hips, butt, thighs and abdomen along with swelling or puffiness in areas like the ankles and fingers points to estrogen dominance. This hormone drives fat storage for child-bearing purposes evolutionarily.

Excess estrogen overwhelms the liver, preventing optimal fat metabolism and causing fluid retention under the skin which gives a puffy appearance.

4. Fatigue, Insomnia and Poor Memory

Excess circulating estrogen and it's metabolites directly impact the brain, worsen inflammation and brain fog. This causes symptoms ranging from debilitating fatigue, difficulty sleeping, mental slowness and memory problems.

Estrogen imbalance combined with inflammation drain mitochondria function. This reduces cellular energy production vital for powering the body and brain optimally through each day.

5. Fertility Issues and Low Libido

Finally, one of the most apparent symptoms tends to be struggling to get pregnant and carry a healthy pregnancy to term. Elevated estrogen hinders ovulation, egg quality, thickens the uterine wall excessively and impedes implantation.

Together with fatigue and mood changes, your sex drive and enjoyment of intimacy often also reduces drastically.

What Causes Estrogen Dominance?

Underlying root causes include:

Imbalanced Stress Hormones

When we face constant high stress levels, this ramps up production of stress hormones like cortisol and adrenaline. Over time, heightened cortisol biases hormonal production towards estrogens through its impact on our endocrine system.

Blood sugar dysregulation due to a high carb, processed food diet also strains the adrenals and stress response.

Obesity and Metabolic Dysfunction

Body fat produces estrogen. So increased fat accumulation specially around the belly and thighs along with insulin resistance activate certain enzymes that convert other hormones like testosterone into estrogen.

The heavier you are, the more estrogen your body will produce from fatty tissue. Losing excess body fat is key.

Nutrient Deficiencies

Lack of key micronutrients like magnesium, B-complex vitamins, vitamin D etc. required for hormone synthesis distorts optimal estrogen metabolism.

These nutrients also combat inflammation and weight gain - both of which fuel estrogen production.

Toxins in Environment and Products

Xenoestrogens are essentially estrogen-mimicking compounds found in plastics, industrial byproducts, pesticides, additives etc. that overexpose our body to excessive estrogenic activity.

Reducing use of products with these toxins as well as good detox habits lower this estrogen burden substantially.

Through the combination of modern high-stress living, poor diet, sedentary lifestyles and environmental pollution, estrogen dominance has become an epidemic for women and men alike.

The downstream effects of the above factors activate a cascade of high estrogen production, inadequate estrogen breakdown, recirculation of used estrogens and widespread estrogenic activity that throws your hormones severely out of balance.

Hope for Healing: The Keys to Balancing Hormones

While complex pathophysiology drives excess estrogen production and reduced progesterone, the good news is that there are concrete steps you can take to reclaim hormonal harmony safely and naturally.

Balancing estrogens requires a holistic multi-modal approach including:

- **Diet and nutrition optimization:** removing inflammatory foods, reducing sugars, ensuring adequate healthy fats and protein, getting key micronutrients etc.

- **Stress management and lifestyle resets:** addressing overwork, lack of sleep, not enough movement or exercise, high alcohol use etc.

- **Targeted nutraceuticals and botanicals:** certain vitamins, minerals, adaptogens, herbs and supplements direct support estrogen metabolism.

- **Reducing external estrogen-like exposures:** minimizing exposure to common xenoestrogens and environmental pollutants.

- **Working with your body's natural cycles:** timing dietary changes, detoxes, supplements etc. align with menstrual phases for gentler continuity.

While symptoms may seem debilitating, trust that your body has a powerful inbuilt capacity to heal and come back into balance when supported properly.

This book provides a comprehensive 28-day plan leveraging evidence-based complementary strategies above to relieve estrogen dominance by addressing root issues holistically.

Chapter 1: Understanding the Estrogen Balance

Estrogen dominance doesn't arise out of the blue. Imbalanced estrogen metabolism is always driven by an intricate interplay of hormonal signals gone awry.

In this chapter, we'll cover the key basics of how estrogen and progesterone function, factors that distort healthy balance leading to estrogen overload along with the downstream impacts.

How Estrogens and Progesterones Work

Estrogens and progesterones are steroid hormones derived primarily from cholesterol. among other key functions, they play an integral role in regulating the menstrual cycle and reproductive health.

The Estrogens

The three major naturally occurring estrogens are estradiol, estriol and estrone:

- Estradiol - Most abundant, potent estrogen
- Estriol - Weaker estrogen produced during pregnancy
- Estrone - Less active estrogen made after menopause

These estrogens exert their effects by binding to estrogen receptors all over the body. Tissues like the uterus, breasts, brain, bone, liver and heart have a high density of these receptors.

The Progesterones

The most important progesterone is Progesterone - the principal progestogen that balances estrogen effects in the body. Other related hormones are testosterone which can convert into estrogen and vice versa depending on enzyme activity.

Cyclical Variations

In women who still have regular periods, both estrogen and progesterone production from the ovaries follows a monthly cyclic pattern:

Follicular Phase: From day 1 of your periods through ovulation, rising estrogen levels stimulate growth of egg follicles and thicken the uterine lining preparing for implantation while keeping progesterone low.

Luteal Phase: Post ovulation, the corpus luteum in the ovary ramps up Progesterone production to balance the estrogen surge. Progesterone primes the cervix, breast tissue etc. for pregnancy.

If no embryo implants, both estrogen and progesterone drop rapidly triggering menstruation and resetting the cycle.

Perimenopausal and postmenopausal individuals see greater fluctuations as ovarian hormone output keeps changing erratically.

Metabolic Pathways

Once produced, estrogens like estradiol undergo extensive liver processing via glucuronidation and hydroxylation into multiple intermediate metabolites before being eliminated from the body.

Healthy metabolism and excretion prevents build-up of used estrogens. Imbalances along the breakdown pathway disrupt this.

Now that we have an overview of hormonal variations, let's look at some key factors that can lead to excess accumulation of estrogens.

Root Causes of Estrogen Dominance

Ovarian Dysfunction

Conditions like PCOS (polycystic ovarian syndrome) hinder ovulation allowing more follicles to remain. These cyst-like follicles produce abnormally high amounts of androgens and estrogens throwing cycles off balance.

Once menopause hits, ovarian shutdown also distorts the estrogen-progesterone equilibrium. Altered body fat distribution results in conversion of additional circulating androgens from the adrenal glands into estrone.

Excess Body Fat

Fat tissue contains an enzyme called aromatase that converts testosterone in the body into estradiol escalating estrogen burden. The more fat you carry, the more substrate exists for estrogen synthesis through this pathway.

Belly and hip fat in particular contribute to elevated estrogen as aromatase activity tends to be higher in these adipose tissue areas.

Chronic Inflammation

Systemic inflammation generates higher levels of an enzyme called COMT which is vital for estrogen breakdown. When

COMT function is impaired via inflammation and oxidative stress, estrogen metabolites recirculate rather than being excreted.

Autoimmunity, food sensitivities, toxins and high stress trigger widespread inflammation making it a pivotal driver.

Nutritional Imbalances

Deficiencies in key micronutrients involved in hormone synthesis like B-vitamins, magnesium, selenium and zinc shift enzymatic activity promoting estrogen dominance.

Excess iron accumulation has also been indicated in distorting hormonal metabolism impacting menstruation. Correcting these inadequacies is vital.

Liver Impairment

Your liver helps filter hormones and produce binding proteins to transport key hormones. Compromised liver function from fatty liver disease, viral infections, alcohol abuse or medication side effects hampers optimal estrogen detoxification.

Liver support is a must in any hormone balancing program.

Toxic Exposure and Endocrine Disruptors

Xenoestrogens are essentially hormone-disrupting estrogen mimics that we ingest through water in plastic bottles, food in plastic containers, conventional body care products, pesticides and many other sources. These drive estrogenic activity and overload.

Now that we have covered the key drivers of excess estrogen, let's look at some vital testing parameters to understand your levels better.

Getting Tested: Understanding Your Hormone Levels

Diagnosing and treating true estrogen dominance requires more nuanced lab testing well beyond a routine annual checkup.

Some key hormones and biomarkers to test for include:

1. Estradiol

Testing specifically blood serum levels of the potent estradiol is preferable over measuring total estrogen that can mask tissue estrogen ratios.

2. Progesterone

Along with Estradiol, assessing progesterone levels is vital to deduce the ratio of estrogen to progesterone. Saliva tests can provide a more real-time indicator than bloodwork.

3. SHBG

Sex hormone binding globulin regulates bioavailability of estrogen. High or low levels impact symptoms drastically despite seemingly normal estrogen.

4. T3 and T4 Thyroid Hormones

Thyroid issues directly worsen estrogen metabolism and exacerbate estrogen overload through crosstalk between pathways. Must be evaluated in tandem.

5. AMH

Anti-mullerian hormone levels can indicate ovarian reserve and guide therapeutics. Checks fertility and perimenopause status.

6. FSH and LH

Follicle stimulating hormone and luteinizing hormone dictate ovarian estrogen production. FSH/LH ratio shifts Signal menopausal stage.

7. Testosterone

Total and free testosterone levels along with DHEAS provide insight on androgen status conversion into estrogen.

8. Vitamin D 25-OH

Low vitamin D correlates strongly with menstrual irregularities, PMS, pain and excess estrogen effects. Quick and easy to assess.

9. hsCRP

High sensitivity C-reactive protein helps quantify inflammatory burden driving estrogen metabolism dysfunction.

Beyond getting the right tests, working with a functional medical practitioner to interpret your symptoms and results in context is invaluable.

Targeted nutritional therapies, stress management, proper liver support and hormone balancing supplements must accompany lifestyle changes to address the root factors we discussed above that are skewing your estrogen levels.

Now that you grasp the key mechanisms of healthy and distorted estrogen balance, let's get into the actionable 28-day healing protocol.

The following chapter provides detailed day-by-day guidelines on dietary recommendations, exercise routines, stress-busting activities, detox protocols and suggested supplements alongside symptom-tracking templates for you to gauge improvements.

Get ready to feel renewed vibrancy, health and wellbeing!

Chapter 2: The 28-Day Plan to Relieve Estrogen Dominance

Welcome to your 28-day healing journey to balance hormones and ease unpleasant estrogen dominance symptoms! In this chapter, we provide a comprehensive, whole-life plan - not just a diet, but a true lifestyle reset to help your body gently return to equilibrium.

We know relief can't come soon enough, but ask you to approach the plan with patience and self-compassion. Lasting balance requires supporting all key organs and systems, reducing exposure to external estrogens and listening closely to your body's innate wisdom.

Here's a quick overview of what you'll find in the 28-day plan:

Diet and Nutrition – Detailed weekly guidelines on foods to embrace and eliminate; meal plans, grocery lists and recipes customized to your menstrual phases to make eating for hormone health simple and satisfying.

Exercise and Lifestyle – Hormone-supportive fitness routines; stress-relieving breathing exercises, meditations and daily self-care rituals to give your adrenals a break from being in overdrive.

Detox and Cleansing - Gentle daily detox practices; guidance on sauna use, dry brushing and natural supplements to clear excess estrogen burden from tissues and support healthy elimination.

Mindset and Tracking - Daily affirmations and mindset practices; symptom tracking templates for you to monitor improvements through the month.

Be flexible! You know your body best, so improvise to adapt protocols to what feels nourishing for you. Temporary detox discomfort often brings the blessing of newfound energy – stick with it!

If you feel unsure or have more significant health issues, work with a functional medicine doctor to customize the plan. Relief IS within reach when we align with nature's rhythms.

Now, let's get started with Week 1! Turn the page for dietary guidelines, meal ideas and more to begin your journey with momentum...

Basic Background Information

Before we dive into the 28-day protocol, let's recap what drives estrogen dominance so you understand exactly why the diet and lifestyle changes are essential.

As covered in Chapter 1, at the root of hormonal chaos lie a few key factors:

Blood Sugar Imbalances – A diet high in refined carbohydrates, sugary foods and insufficient protein spikes insulin and disrupts endocrine function. Stable blood sugar and insulin sensitivity form the foundation of any hormone balancing effort.

Gut Health – Chronic inflammation and infection in the GI tract hampers estrogen detoxification through the liver – your main pathway for estrogen metabolism and elimination.

Healing foods, gut-friendly herbs and probiotic supplementation can help transform gut environment.

Toxic Burden – Accumulation of xenoestrogens from environment/products and inadequate elimination of these mimics contributes to high circulating estrogen levels. Minimizing exposure plus supporting detox organs can alleviate this burden.

Nutritional Deficiencies – Lack of key micronutrients for optimal steroid hormone synthesis like magnesium, B vitamins, vitamin D allows estrogen/progesterone imbalance to persist. A micronutrient-dense diet is crucial.

Chronic Stress – High daily stress levels lead to elevated cortisol production, which biases the body towards churning out more estrogen and disrupts endocrine feedback loops. Stress management is critical for lasting balance.

Liver Health – A sluggish liver fails to properly filter hormones and facilitate estrogen breakdown into benign metabolites for safe elimination from your body. Enhancing liver function enables estrogen detox.

The exact mix of factors above are unique for each woman. But employing a comprehensive strategy that addresses all of them is key to long-term relief.

The integrative protocols covered over the next 28 days leverage natural mechanisms in the body to heal and come back into equilibrium when supported properly. Think of it as working *with* your body's innate intelligence rather than forcing change or deprivation from the outside.

Let's get you started! On the next page we start guiding you through the week-by-week plan, with meal ideas, lifestyle tips and supplement recommendations specially designed for your first 7 days of this journey back to feeling healthy and vibrant.

Week 1

Congratulations on embarking on your healing journey! Week 1 focuses on removing pro-inflammatory foods that disrupt hormonal pathways, nutrient-dense ingredients to correct deficiencies, and initiating gentle liver detoxification for laying the foundation before we add in more targeted hormone balancing interventions in later weeks.

Your Week 1 Guidelines:

Diet:

- Remove gluten, dairy, soy, corn, pork, alcohol and caffeine
- Focus on organic vegetables, fruits, clean proteins and healthy fats
- Drink lemon water first thing in the morning to stimulate liver detoxification
- Herbal detox tea before bed
- Take 1 Tbsp apple cider vinegar before larger carb-heavy meals to blunt blood sugar spikes

Nutrient-Dense Ingredients to Emphasize:

- Cruciferous vegetables: broccoli, kale, Brussels sprouts, cabbage etc.
- Starchy tubers: sweet potato, yam, potato

- Anti-inflammatory fats: Avocado, coconut oil, ghee, nut oils

- Clean proteins: Fatty fish, pasture-raised poultry and eggs

- Soaked/sprouted nuts and seeds

- Berries and low glycemic index fruit: blueberries, raspberries etc.

Lifestyle:

- 10-15 minute morning meditation session

- 5 minute hourly movement breaks

- 8-9 hours nightly sleep aiming for before 10pm bedtime

Supplements:

- Start taking a high quality probiotic 20-30 billion CFUs

- 1000-2000mg Omega 3 fish oils for anti-inflammatory benefits

- Vitamin C - 500mg twice daily to support liver pathways

- B-complex vitamin to cover any nutritional gaps

Shopping List for Week 1:

- Pasture raised eggs

- Mixed greens

- Cruciferous vegetables

- Fresh wild caught salmon
- Bone broth collagen powder
- Low sugar nut milk
- Fresh or frozen organic berries
- Sweet potato
- Avocado oil
- Apple cider vinegar
- Lemons
- B-complex vitamin
- Probiotic supplement
- Omega 3 fish oil

Week 1 Meal Plan and Recipes

Day 1

Breakfast:

Veggie Frittata

- 6 eggs
- 1/2 onion, diced
- 1 cup baby spinach
- 1/2 cup cherry tomatoes, halved
- 1/4 cup feta cheese

- Whisk eggs in a bowl, season with salt and pepper.
- Sauté onion and spinach.
- Pour eggs into pan, top with tomatoes.
- Sprinkle feta cheese.
- Bake at 350°F for 20 minutes until set.

Lunch:

Massaged Kale Salad

- 4 cups kale, ribs removed and chopped
- 1/4 cup extra virgin olive oil
- 2 tbsp lemon juice
- 1 avocado, diced
- 1/2 cup chickpeas
- Baked salmon fillet
- Massage kale with olive oil and lemon juice.
- Top with chickpeas, avocado, salmon.

Dinner:

Chicken Soup

- 8 cups bone broth
- 1 lb boneless chicken breasts
- 2 carrots, chopped

- 2 stalks celery, chopped
- 1 sweet potato, chopped
- 1 tbsp collagen peptides
- Bring broth to a boil in a pot.
- Add chicken, carrots, celery and sweet potato.
- Simmer for 20 minutes.
- Remove chicken and shred, return to pot
- Stir in collagen peptides before serving.

Day 2

Breakfast:

Berry Protein Smoothie

- 1 cup nut milk
- 1/2 cup frozen mixed berries
- 1 scoop vanilla plant-based protein powder
- 1 tbsp almond butter
- 1 tsp flaxseed
- Blend all ingredients until smooth.

Lunch:

Grilled Veg Wrap

- 1 large whole grain wrap

- 1/2 cup mixed grilled veggies
- Hummus
- Lettuce
- Spread hummus on wrap.
- Top with grilled veggies and lettuce.

Dinner:

Sheet Pan Lemony Fish & Veggies

- 1 lb cod fillets
- 2 cups green beans
- Cherry tomatoes
- 1 lemon
- 2 tbsp olive oil
- Toss veggies with oil, lemon juice, salt & pepper.
- Roast veggies for 10 minutes on a sheet pan.
- Push veggies to edges, add fish to center.
- Roast 5-10 more mins until fish flakes.

Day 3

Breakfast:

Breakfast Hash

- 2 eggs

- 1/2 cup sweet potato, diced 1/2"
- 1/2 onion, diced
- 1 cup spinach
- 1/4 cup black beans
- Over medium heat, sauté sweet potato and onion 5 minutes
- Add spinach and beans, cook 1 minute more.
- Make two wells, crack an egg into each, season.
- Cover and cook 5-7 minutes until eggs reach desired doneness.

Lunch:

Lentil & Quinoa Bowl

- 1/2 cup cooked quinoa
- 1/2 cup cooked lentils
- 1 cup mixed greens
- 1/4 avocado, sliced
- 2 tbsp Tahini dressing
- Divide quinoa, lentils, greens between two bowls
- Top with avocado and drizzle with dressing

Dinner:

Sheet Pan Lemon Garlic Salmon

- 2 salmon fillets
- 2 tbsp olive oil
- 4 garlic cloves, minced
- 1 lemon
- Asparagus
- Toss asparagus in 1 tbsp oil, season with salt & pepper
- Roast at 400°F for 5 minutes on sheet pan
- Push asparagus to edges, place salmon in center
- Sprinkle salmon generously with minced garlic
- Squeeze lemon juice over salmon
- Roast 8-10 minutes until salmon flakes apart

Day 4

Breakfast:

Veggie Omelet

- 3 eggs
- 1/4 onion, diced
- 1/2 cup spinach
- 2 mushrooms, sliced
- 1/4 cup cheddar
- Whisk eggs with salt and pepper
- Pour eggs into oiled hot pan

- Top one half with onion, spinach, mushrooms
- When bottom sets, fold empty half over filling
- Sprinkle cheddar, cover to melt 1-2 minutes

Lunch:

Chicken & Quinoa Salad

- 3 oz baked chicken, shredded
- 1/2 cup cooked quinoa
- 1/2 apple, diced
- 1 stalk celery, diced
- 2 tbsp balsamic dressing
- Combine chicken, quinoa, apple and celery
- Add balsamic dressing, toss to coat

Dinner:

Veggie & Tofu Stir Fry

- 1 cup broccoli florets
- 1 red pepper, sliced
- 8 oz firm tofu, cubed
- 2 tbsp coconut oil
- 2 garlic cloves, minced
- 2 tbsp stir fry sauce

- Heat 1 tbsp oil in a pan. Add tofu, cook 5 minutes
- Remove tofu, heat remaining oil
- Stir fry garlic for 1 minute
- Add broccoli & pepper, cook 5 minutes
- Return tofu to pan with stir fry sauce

Day 5

Breakfast:

Ham & Cheese Egg Cups

- 6 eggs
- 1/4 cup diced ham
- 1/4 cup shredded cheddar cheese
- Salt and pepper
- Grease a muffin tin with oil or line with cups
- Whisk eggs and seasonings, stir in ham and cheese
- Distribute evenly into cups
- Bake at 350°F for 15-20 minutes until set

Lunch:

Loaded Baked Sweet Potato

- 1 medium sweet potato
- 1/4 cup black beans

- 1/4 avocado, mashed
- 2 tbsp Greek yogurt
- 1 tbsp hot sauce
- Bake sweet potato at 400°F 45-60 minutes until tender
- Slice open and mash flesh, top with remaining ingredients

Dinner:

Pesto Chicken Pasta

- 8 oz gluten-free pasta
- 2 cups kale, chopped
- 1 lb chicken, cooked and shredded
- 1/4 cup pesto
- Juice from 1 lemon
- Cook pasta according to package instructions
- In the last two minutes add the kale to blanch
- Drain and transfer to a large bowl
- Add chicken, pesto and lemon juice - toss to combine

Day 6

Breakfast:

Berry Banana Protein Smoothie

- 1 banana, frozen

- 1 cup kale or spinach leaves
- 1 cup nut milk
- 1/2 cup mixed berries
- 2 tbsp hemp seeds
- 1 scoop vanilla protein powder
- Add all ingredients into high powered blender
- Blend until smooth and creamy texture is reached

Lunch:

Buckwheat Soba Noodle Salad

- 4 oz buckwheat soba noodles, cooked
- 1 cup shredded purple cabbage
- 1 red pepper, sliced
- 1/4 cup chopped cilantro
- 1 tbsp sesame oil
- 3 tbsp peanut sauce
- In a bowl combine the noodles, vegetables and cilantro
- Toss with sesame oil, peanut sauce and a squeeze of lime juice

Dinner:

Sheet Pan Ginger Salmon

- 2 salmon fillets
- 2 cups green beans
- 2 cups broccoli florets
- 1 tbsp olive oil
- 1 tbsp minced ginger
- 2 garlic cloves, minced
- Toss veggies with olive oil, minced ginger and garlic
- Roast veggies at 400°F for 5 minutes on a sheet pan
- Push veggies to edges, place salmon in center
- Roast 8-12 minutes until veggies tender and salmon flakes apart

Day 7
Breakfast:

Breakfast Tacos

- 6 eggs
- 1/2 onion, diced
- 1 tomato, diced
- 1 avocado
- Salsa
- 4 taco-size tortillas
- Whisk eggs in bowl with a splash of milk or water

- Pour eggs into hot pan with oil, let set slightly
- Stir in onions and tomatoes
- Warm tortillas; fill with egg mixture and salsa, top with avocado

Lunch:

Chicken Caesar Salad

- 5 oz baked chicken breast, sliced
- 4 cups romaine lettuce, chopped
- 1/4 cup parmesan cheese
- 2-3 tbsp caesar dressing
- On a plate or in a shallow bowl, layer lettuce leaves
- Top with sliced chicken and parmesan cheese
- Drizzle caesar dressing over salad

Dinner:

Zoodles with Shrimp

- 4 zucchini, spiralized into noodles
- 1 tbsp olive oil
- 12 large shrimp, peeled
- 2 garlic cloves, minced
- 1 cup cherry tomatoes, halved
- 1/4 cup basil leaves, chopped

- 2 tbsp Parmesan cheese
- Heat olive oil in a skillet over medium heat.
- Cook shrimp and garlic for 3 minutes, stirring frequently.
- Add zucchini noodles and continue cooking for 4 more minutes until tender but still crisp.
- Remove from heat and stir in tomatoes, basil and parmesan. Enjoy!

Wishing you bountiful energy as you kickstart your journey into renewed hormonal health and vitality this week! Keep turning the page for Week 1 recipes...

Week 2

Fantastic job completing Week 1! Let's keep up the momentum.

Week 2 builds on the foundation by doubling down on liver support, estrogen metabolism and gut healing foods while reintroducing non-inflammatory grains, legumes and animal proteins in moderation.

Your Week 2 Guidelines:

Diet:

- Reintroduce gluten-free whole grains like brown rice, buckwheat, millet
- Incorporate legumes: lentils, chickpeas, peas, beans
- Organic corn tortillas ok in moderation

- Limit animal protein to 12-16 oz per day
- Continue avoiding gluten, dairy, soy, caffeine

Nutrient-Dense Foods to Emphasize:

- Beets - phytonutrients enhance estrogen breakdown
- Cruciferous veggies - contain DIM and IC3 to facilitate elimination
- Onions/garlic - sulfur compounds aid liver detox
- Pears/apples - fiber prevents estrogen reabsorption
- Flax/chia - lignans block estrogen receptors

Lifestyle:

- Begin 15-20 min HIIT workouts 2 x week
- Start dry brushing before showering
- Schedule sauna sessions if possible
- Stretching before bed

Supplements:

- Milk thistle or SAMe to enhance liver function
- Calcium d-glucarate - binds "used" estrogens for excretion
- Continue probiotic, omega 3, B-complex and Vitamin C

Shopping List for Week 2:

- Beets + beet greens

- Cruciferous vegetables
- Onions/Garlic
- Bell peppers
- Quinoa/brown rice
- Chickpeas and lentils
- Pears or green apples
- Flax seeds/chia seeds
- Milk thistle supplements
- Calcium d-glucarate

Week 2 Meal Plan and Recipes

Day 1

Breakfast:

Beet Green Smoothie

- 1 cup beet greens
- 1 small beet, chopped
- 1 banana
- 1 cup nut milk
- 1/2 cup Greek yogurt
- 1 tbsp chia seeds
- 1/2 tsp cinnamon

- Blend all ingredients in blender until smooth.

Lunch:

Chickpea Zucchini Fritters

- 1 15oz can chickpeas, drained and mashed
- 1 zucchini, shredded
- 1 egg
- 1/4 cup almond flour
- 1 tsp cumin
- 1 garlic clove, minced
- Mix mashed chickpeas with remaining ingredients.
- Form into patties and pan fry in oil 3-4 minutes per side.
- Serve on top of salad.

Dinner:

Veggie Quinoa Stuffed Pepper

- 1 red bell pepper, tops cut off
- 1/2 cup cooked quinoa
- 1/2 cup black beans
- 1 cup roasted broccoli
- 1/4 cup salsa
- Mix quinoa, beans, broccoli and salsa.

- Stuff pepper with quinoa mixture and bake 25 minutes at 375°F.

Day 2

Breakfast:

Green Goddess Smoothie

- 2 cups spinach
- 1 pear, sliced
- 1 cup nut milk
- 1/2 avocado
- 1 tbsp honey
- Blend until smooth.

Lunch:

Lentil Pita Pockets

- Whole grain pita bread, halved
- Lentils
- Lettuce, tomato, onion
- Tzatziki sauce
- Spread tzatziki in pitas, stuff with lentils, veggies.

Dinner:

Sheet Pan Lemon Chicken & Asparagus

- Chicken breasts

- Asparagus, olive oil, salt
- Lemon wedges
- Bake chicken and asparagus in sheet pan at 400°F 15 minutes.
- Squeeze lemon juice on chicken.

Day 3

Breakfast:

Breakfast Rice Pudding

- 1/2 cup brown rice, cooked
- 1 cup almond milk
- 1/4 cup raisins
- Cinnamon
- Maple syrup
- Simmer rice in milk 5 minutes.
- Stir in raisins, cinnamon and syrup.

Lunch:

Chickpea Salad Sandwich

- 1 15oz can chickpeas, drained
- 1/4 cup vegan mayo
- Celery, onion, pickles
- 2 slices whole grain bread

- Mash chickpeas with mayo, diced veggies.
- Spread on bread, enjoy open-faced.

Dinner:

One Pan Chicken & Rice

- Chicken breast, diced
- 1 cup brown rice
- Broccoli florets
- Garlic, avocado oil
- Sauté chicken 3 minutes in oil.
- Add rice, broccoli, garlic.
- Cook covered 20 minutes until done.

Day 4

Breakfast:

Veggie Egg Muffins

- 6 eggs, beaten
- Spinach, tomato, onion
- Feta cheese
- Grease muffin tin, pour in egg mixture with veggies.
- Sprinkle feta cheese, bake 20 minutes.

Lunch:

Mason Jar Chopped Salad

- Mixed greens
- Quinoa
- Carrots
- Chickpeas
- Ranch dressing
- Layer salad ingredients in mason jar.
- Shake/mix together when ready to eat.

Dinner:

Sheet Pan Fajitas

- Flank steak
- Onion, bell pepper
- Corn tortillas
- Guacamole etc.
- Roast veggies and steak 15 mins at 400°F.
- Serve in tortillas with desired toppings.

Day 5

Breakfast:

Apple Cinnamon Oatmeal

- 1/2 cup oats

- 1 cup almond milk
- 1 apple, diced
- cinnamon, honey
- Cook oats in milk.
- Stir in apple, cinnamon and honey.

Lunch:

Lentil & Kale Soup

- Lentils, kale, carrots, celery
- 32oz broth
- Lemon juice
- Simmer lentil and veggies in broth 20 minutes.
- Finish with lemon juice.

Dinner:

Quinoa Buddha Bowl

- Quinoa
- Roasted veggies
- Avocado
- Tofu, cashews
- Prepare bowl with quinoa base and pile on desired toppings.

Day 6

Breakfast:

Breakfast Tacos

- Eggs
- Bell pepper, onion
- Salsa
- Corn tortillas
- Scramble pepper, onion, eggs in pan.
- Serve in warm tortillas with salsa.

Lunch:

Grilled Chicken & Pear Salad

- Mixed greens
- Chicken breast
- Pears, feta cheese
- Balsamic dressing
- Assemble salad ingredients, drizzle with dressing.

Dinner:

Eggplant & Bean Casserole

- Eggplant, onion, garlic
- White beans
- Marinara sauce

- Cheese (optional)
- Layer sliced eggplant with beans, sauce in baking dish.
- Bake 30 minutes at 350°F until hot and bubbly.

Day 7

Breakfast:

Overnight Chia Oats

- 1/2 cup oats
- 1 cup almond milk
- 2 tbsp chia seeds
- Berries, honey to taste
- Mix everything (except berries & honey), refrigerate overnight.
- Top with berries & honey before eating.

Lunch:

Superfood Collard Wraps

- Collard greens
- Quinoa
- Avocado
- Carrots
- Tahini dressing

- Softens collard leaves by blanching or microwaving briefly.
- Fill leaves with quinoa mixture and dressing. Roll up.

Dinner:

Roasted Salmon

- Salmon fillets
- Broccoli
- Brown rice
- Lemon
- Roast salmon and broccoli at 400°F 15 minutes.
- Serve over brown rice with lemon.

Track any symptoms this week and let me know how the plan is working for you!

Week 3

We're halfway through! Let's keep the momentum going strong in week 3.

This week, we introduce metabolism and hormone balancing superfoods, bitters to stimulate digestion plus begin intermittent fasting to give the liver extended breaks for enhanced cellular repair and detoxification.

Your Week 3 Guidelines:

Diet:

- Add omega-3 rich seafood 2-3 times per week
- Incorporate metabolism boosting spices - turmeric, cinnamon, oregano
- Raw cacao nibs for antioxidant and magnesium benefits
- Begin 16-hour intermittent fasts twice weekly
- Have a cup of warm lemon water with 5-10 drops of bitters upon waking to stimulate bile flow

Nutrient-Dense Foods to Emphasize:

- Wild-caught salmon and sardines
- Leafy greens - nettle, dandelion, kale
- Cruciferous veggies continued
- Berries packed with antioxidants
- Avocado for healthy fats
- Chia, hemp and flax seeds

Lifestyle:

- Continue HIIT workouts 2-3 times weekly
- Extend nightly fast to 12 hours
- Alternate hot and cold showers
- Schedule reflexology session

Supplements:

- DIM or I3C capsules to facilitate estrogen metabolism

- Milk thistle or liver support herbal blend continued
- Vitex to help rebalance hormonal equilibrium
- Magnesium transdermal spray before bed

Shopping List for Week 3:

- Wild-caught salmon and halibut
- Assorted berries
- Spinach and mixed greens
- Cruciferous veggies
- Chia, flax and hemp seeds
- Bitters tinctures
- DIM/I3C and vitex supplements

Week 3 Meal Plan and Recipes

Day 1

Breakfast:

Lox Stacked Toast

- 2 slices sprouted grain bread
- 2 oz smoked salmon
- 1 oz cream cheese
- 1 tomato, sliced
- Capers, red onion

- Toast bread. Spread cream cheese.
- Top with lox, tomato, capers, onion

Lunch:

Cranberry Spinach Salad

- Baby spinach leaves
- 1/4 red onion, sliced
- 1/4 cup dried cranberries
- 1 avocado, cubed
- 2 tbsp balsamic vinaigrette
- In a salad bowl, combine spinach, cranberries, onion, avocado
- Drizzle with balsamic vinaigrette

Dinner:

Lemon Herb Baked Halibut

- 1 lb halibut fillets
- 2 tbsp olive oil
- 2 garlic cloves, minced
- 1 lemon
- 1 tsp oregano
- Place halibut in baking dish, drizzle oil

- Squeeze lemon juice over top and sprinkle garlic and oregano
- Bake at 400°F 15 mins until fish flakes easily with fork

Day 2

Breakfast:

Overnight Oats

- 1/2 cup oats
- 1 cup almond milk
- 1 tbsp chia seeds
- 1/2 cup mixed berries
- Combine oats, milk, chia in jar. Refrigerate overnight.
- Top with berries before eating.

Lunch:

Chickpea Avocado Salad Sandwich

- 1 can chickpeas, rinsed and drained
- 1 avocado, mashed
- 1 tbsp vegan mayo
- 1 celery stalk, finely diced
- 2 slices Ezekiel bread
- In bowl, mix chickpeas with mayo, avocado and celery

- Spread between bread slices

Dinner:

Pistachio Crusted Salmon

- 2 salmon fillets
- 2 tbsp pistachio nuts, crushed
- 2 tbsp paprika
- 2 tbsp olive oil
- Coat salmon fillets with combined pistachio crumbs and paprika
- Place on baking sheet and drizzle with olive oil
- Bake at 400°F for 12-15 mins until flaky

Day 3

Breakfast:

Spinach & Tomato Frittata

- 6 eggs, beaten
- 1 cup spinach, chopped
- 1 tomato, diced
- 2 oz feta cheese
- Preheat oven to 375°F.
- Combine eggs, spinach, tomato, salt and pepper in bowl

- Pour into oiled baking dish, sprinkle feta on top
- Bake 20 minutes until set

Lunch:

Mediterranean Chickpea Mason Jar Salad

- Chickpeas
- Cucumber, tomatoes, olives
- Romaine lettuce leaves
- Lemon vinaigrette
- Layer salad ingredients in jar in order
- Shake/mix ingredients together when ready to eat

Dinner:

Pan-Seared Cod with Herb Sauce

- 4 cod fillets
- 1 lemon
- Small bunch parsley
- 1 garlic clove
- 1/4 cup olive oil
- Squeeze lemon juice into blender, add parsley, garlic and olive oil. Blend.
- Pat cod dry, season, and pan-sear. Serve with herb sauce.

Day 4

Breakfast:

Green Protein Smoothie

- 1 cup almond milk
- 1/2 cup spinach
- 1/2 avocado
- 1/2 cup green grapes
- 1 scoop protein powder
- Blend all ingredients until smooth

Lunch:

Egg Salad Lettuce Wraps

- 4 hard boiled eggs, chopped
- 1 celery stalk, diced
- 1 tbsp olive oil mayo
- Boston lettuce leaves
- Gently mix eggs, celery and mayo
- Scoop mixture into lettuce leaf and wrap

Dinner:

Pesto Zucchini Noodles with Shrimp

- 3 small zucchini, spiralized

- 12 large shrimp, tails removed
- 2 cups cherry tomatoes, halved
- 1/4 cup pesto
- Saute zucchini noodles for 2-3 mins until slightly softened
- Add shrimp and cherry tomatoes. Cook until shrimp is pink. Remove from heat and stir in pesto.

Day 5

Breakfast:

Sweet Potato Hash with Eggs

- 1 sweet potato, diced
- 1/2 bell pepper, diced
- 1/2 onion, diced
- Olive oil
- Salt & pepper
- 2 eggs
- Heat oil in skillet over medium heat. Add potatoes, pepper and onion with seasonings. Cook for 15 minutes, flipping occasionally.
- Make two wells, crack eggs into them. Cover and cook until desired donencss.

Lunch:

Mediterranean Tuna Salad

- 1 can tuna, drained
- 1/4 cucumber, diced
- 4 cherry tomatoes, quartered
- 1/4 cup black olives, sliced
- 2 tbsp olive oil
- 1 tbsp red wine vinegar
- Lettuce leaves
- In a bowl, combine tuna, cucumber, tomatoes and olives.
- Whisk together oil and vinegar, drizzle over salad.
- Serve tuna salad over lettuce leaves.

Dinner:

Lemon Garlic Shrimp Skewers

- 12 large shrimp
- Wooden skewers
- 2 lemons, juiced
- 4 garlic cloves, minced
- 2 tbsp olive oil
- In bowl, combine lemon juice, garlic and olive oil. Add shrimp and let marinate 10 minutes.

- Skewer shrimp. Grill or broil 3 minutes per side until cooked through.

Day 6

Breakfast:

Tropical Acai Bowl

- 1 pack Sambazon organic acai smoothie pack
- 1 banana, sliced
- 1/2 cup pineapple chunks
- 1/4 cup granola
- Blend smoothie packet with banana, 1 cup water and pineapple.
- Top with granola.

Lunch:

Lentil Walnut Lettuce Cups

- Cooked brown lentils
- Diced red onion
- Chopped walnuts
- Lemon juice
- Lettuce leaves
- Gently mix lentils, walnuts, onion. Add lemon juice and season.
- Divide mixture among lettuce cups.

Dinner:

Broiled Lemon & Herb Whitefish

- 1 lb whitefish fillets
- 1 lemon, thinly sliced
- 1/4 cup fresh parsley
- 2 tbsp olive oil
- Salt & pepper to taste
- Arrange fillets in baking dish. Layer lemon slices on top and scatter parsley.
- Drizzle with olive oil and season.
- Broil 8-10 minutes until fish is opaque and cooked through.

Day 7

Breakfast:

Berry Almond Smoothie Bowl

- 1 cup almond milk
- 1 cup frozen mixed berries
- 2 scoops protein powder
- Toppings: Granola, almonds, hemp seeds
- Blend almond milk, berries and protein powder.
- Pour into a bowl, top with mix-ins.

Lunch:

Egg Salad Collard Green Wrap

- 4 hardboiled eggs, chopped
- 1 celery stalk, minced
- 1/4 cup plain Greek yogurt
- 2 large collard green leaves
- Stir together eggs, celery, yogurt, salt & pepper.
- Spoon mixture onto collard green leaves, wrap and enjoy.

Dinner:

Sheet Pan Teriyaki Salmon Bowls

- 4 salmon fillets
- 1 lb broccoli florets
- 1 cup quinoa
- Teriyaki sauce
- Arrange salmon and broccoli on a sheet pan. Drizzle teriyaki sauce. Bake at 400°F 15 mins.
- Divide cooked quinoa between bowls, top with salmon and broccoli.

You got this! Keep up the phenomenal efforts nourishing your body and mind.

Week 4

We've made it to the final week of the program! You should be feeling incredibly proud of the dedication you've shown your body. Let's finish strong and set you up for continued success.

Week 4 solidifies the diet and lifestyle changes that support healthy estrogen metabolism while beginning to loosen some restrictions now that detox pathways are primed. We also provide guidance on transitioning smoothly back to a sustainable nutrition plan tailored to your unique needs.

Your Week 4 Guidelines:

Diet:

- Reintroduce gluten-free whole grains like brown rice and millet
- Legumes and lentils continue to be encouraged
- Minimal amounts of grass-fed dairy permitted
- Limit red meat intake to 1-2 times weekly
- Cold-water, low mercury fish options still emphasized

Nutrient-Dense Foods to Emphasize:

- Cruciferous vegetables
- Berries high in antioxidants
- Bone broth for collagen, amino acids
- Turmeric, ginger, garlic and oregano
- Good fats - avocado, seeds/nuts, olive oil

Lifestyle:
- Ongoing HIIT workouts
- Additional supplements based on symptoms
- Begin drafting post detox eating plan
- Practice mindfulness and self-care rituals

Supplements:
- Liver support nutrients like milk thistle
- DIM or I3C for healthy estrogen metabolism
- Vitex cycle-support
- Magnesium, zinc and B-vitamins as needed

Shopping List for Week 4:
- Eggs, Cod, Lentils
- Bell peppers, Broccoli, Spinach
- Blueberries, Avocado
- Bone broth, Olive oil, Apple cider vinegar
- Turmeric, Garlic, Ginger, Oregano

Week 4 Meal Plan and Recipes

Day 1

Breakfast:

Veggie Scrambled Eggs

- 6 eggs
- 1 cup baby spinach, chopped
- 1/4 cup cherry tomatoes, diced
- 2 tbsp feta cheese, crumbled
- Whisk eggs in a bowl, season with salt and pepper.
- Pour eggs into a pan with oil over medium heat.
- Add spinach and tomatoes, stir frequently 3-5 minutes until eggs are set but still moist.
- Remove from heat, sprinkle with feta.

Lunch:

Lentil Walnut Stuffed Pepper

- 1 red bell pepper, tops and seeds removed
- 1 cup cooked lentils
- 1/4 cup walnuts, chopped
- 1 garlic clove, minced
- 2 cups baby spinach
- Preheat oven to 375°F. In a bowl, mix filling ingredients.
- Stuff pepper with lentil mixture and place on a baking sheet or casserole dish.
- Bake 25 minutes until pepper is tender.

Dinner:

Miso Glazed Cod

- 4 cod fillets (5-6 oz each)
- 3 tbsp white miso paste
- 1 tbsp pure maple syrup
- 2 tsp Dijon mustard
- 1 garlic clove, grated
- Mix the miso, maple syrup, mustard and garlic together in a shallow dish. Add cod fillets and turn to coat both sides.
- Roast at 425°F for 12 minutes until cod flakes easily with a fork.

Day 2

Breakfast:

Blueberry Pecan Oatmeal

- 1/2 cup steel cut oats
- 1 cup almond milk
- 1/4 cup pecans, chopped
- 1/2 cup blueberries
- Bring oats and milk to a boil, then reduce heat. Simmer 10 minutes, stirring occasionally until thick and creamy.
- Remove from heat, stir in pecans and blueberries.

Lunch:

Mediterranean Chickpea Mason Jar Salad

- 1 cup cooked chickpeas
- Diced cucumber, tomatoes, red onion
- 2 cups mixed greens
- 2 tbsp balsamic vinaigrette
- Layer the salad ingredients neatly in a jar in order.
- Shake vigorously when ready to eat to mix things up.

Dinner:

Green Bean Almondine Salmon

- 4 salmon fillets
- 1 lb green beans, ends trimmed
- 1/4 cup toasted sliced almonds
- Zest and juice from 1 lemon
- Roast salmon skin-side down with green beans tossed in oil at 400°F for 12-15 minutes until cooked through and tender.
- Transfer salmon and green beans to plates, top with almonds. Squeeze lemon juice over.

Day 3

Breakfast:

Avocado Bacon Deviled Eggs

- 6 hard boiled eggs, halved lengthwise
- 1 avocado, mashed
- 2 slices cooked turkey bacon, crumbled
- 1 tbsp Greek yogurt
- Smoked paprika, salt & pepper
- Scoop yolks into bowl, mash smooth with a fork.
- Stir in mashed avocado, bacon crumbles, yogurt and spices.
- Spoon or pipe filling back into egg whites.

Lunch:

Curried Chickpea Salad Sandwich

- 1 can chickpeas, drained and rinsed
- 1/4 cup plain Greek yogurt
- 1 celery stalk, diced
- 1 tsp curry powder
- 1 tbsp lemon juice
- 2 slices sprouted bread
- Mash chickpeas into a chunky paste. Stir in remaining ingredients except bread slices.
- Spread chickpea salad onto bread and enjoy.

Dinner:

Sheet Pan Teriyaki Chicken

- 2 boneless skinless chicken breasts, cubed
- 1 crown broccoli, cut into florets
- Sweet potato, peeled and diced
- 3 tbsp teriyaki sauce
- Toss chicken and veggies with teriyaki sauce on a baking sheet.
- Roast at 425°F for 20 minutes until chicken is cooked through.

Day 4

Breakfast:

Coconut Chia Seed Pudding

- 1 (14 oz) can coconut milk
- 1/3 cup chia seeds
- 1 tsp vanilla extract
- Fresh berries
- Whisk together coconut milk, chia seeds and vanilla in a bowl. Refrigerate overnight or at least 2 hours.
- Serve chilled sprinkled with berries.

Lunch:

Leftover Lentil Walnut Stuffed Pepper

Dinner:

Sheet Pan Honey Lime Tilapia

- 4 tilapia fillets
- 2 bell peppers, sliced
- 2 zucchinis, sliced
- 2 limes, juiced
- 2 tbsp olive oil
- 2 tbsp honey
- Toss veggies with oil on sheet pan, air fry/roast 10 minutes at 400°F.
- Push veggies to edges, add tilapia to center. Squeeze lime juice and drizzle honey over fish.
- Roast 10 more minutes until opaque and veggies are tender.

Day 5

Breakfast:

Veggie Egg White Scramble

- 6 egg whites
- 1/2 cup mushrooms, sliced
- 1/4 cup cherry tomatoes, quartered

- Spinach leaves
- 1 oz feta cheese
- Spray pan with oil and saute mushrooms and tomatoes over medium heat 3 minutes.
- Add egg whites, scramble until set but still moist, 3-4 minutes.
- Serve over a bed of spinach, topped with crumbled feta.

Lunch:

Italian Tuna Lettuce Wraps

- 1 can tuna packed in olive oil
- Artichoke hearts from jar, chopped
- Sundried tomatoes, chopped
- 1 tbsp balsamic glaze
- Romaine lettuce leaves
- Gently mix tuna, artichokes and tomatoes in a bowl. Drizzle over balsamic glaze.
- Scoop tuna mixture into romaine lettuce leaf cups.

Dinner:

Sheet Pan Lemon Garlic Salmon & Broccoli

- 2 salmon fillets

- 4 cups broccoli florets
- 2 tbsp olive oil
- 4 cloves garlic, minced
- Zest and juice from 1 lemon
- Toss broccoli and oil, spread on baking sheet pan.
- Place salmon in the middle, sprinkle generously with minced garlic.
- Broil 8-12 minutes until fish flakes and broccoli tender.
- Finish with lemon zest and fresh lemon juice.

Day 6

Breakfast:

Apple Pie Chia Seed Pudding

- 1 cup almond milk
- 1/3 cup chia seeds
- 1 apple, grated
- 1 tsp cinnamon
- 1 tsp vanilla extract
- Maple syrup to taste
- Stir together all ingredients except maple syrup. Refrigerate overnight.
- Top servings with maple syrup before eating.

Lunch:

Mediterranean Chickpea Quinoa Salad

- 1 cup cooked quinoa
- 1 can chickpeas, drained and rinsed
- Diced tomatoes, cucumbers, red onion
- Crumbled feta cheese
- Fresh herbs
- Red wine vinegar
- In a large bowl, combine cooked quinoa, chickpeas and vegetables.
- In a small bowl, whisk vinegar and olive oil. Pour over salad, then mix in feta and herbs.

Dinner:

Green Goddess Salmon Burgers

- 1 lb salmon, chopped
- 1/2 cup bread crumbs
- 1 egg
- 2 garlic cloves
- 3 tbsp parsley
- Lemon juice
- Pulse salmon, breadcrumbs, egg and garlic in food processor until combined but still chunky.

- Form into patties, pan fry until browned and opaque throughout, 4-5 mins per side.
- Mix parsley and lemon juice, serve salmon cakes with green goddess sauce.

Day 7

Breakfast:

Veggie Egg Bake

- 6 eggs
- 3 egg whites
- Chopped broccoli, tomatoes, spinach
- Shredded cheddar cheese
- Beat eggs and egg whites, pour into greased casserole dish.
- Mix in chopped vegetables and top with shredded cheese.
- Bake at 375 degrees for 30 minutes until set. Let stand 5 minutes before cutting.

Lunch:

Mediterranean Baked Sweet Potato

- 1 large sweet potato
- Roasted red peppers
- Crumbled feta

- Kalamata olives
- Red onion
- Fresh oregano
- Bake sweet potato until tender, cut down the center.
- Top with remaining ingredients.

Dinner:

Sheet Pan Apricot Glazed Pork Tenderloin

- 1 lb pork tenderloin
- 10 oz Brussels sprouts, halved
- 2 tbsp olive oil
- 1/4 cup apricot jam
- 2 tbsp balsamic vinegar
- 1 garlic clove, minced
- Toss brussels sprouts with 1 tbsp oil on baking sheet. Roast at 400°F for 5 minutes.
- In a bowl, mix jam, vinegar, garlic and remaining 1 tbsp oil. Rub mixture evenly over pork.
- Push sprouts to one side and put pork on other side of sheet.
- Roast 15 minutes more until pork reaches 145°F internally and sprouts are caramelized.

You made it! Trust all the positive dietary and lifestyle changes you've implemented will continue serving you long beyond the 28 days.

Beyond Food: Additional Protocols

While diet provides the strong foundation, complementary detox and lifestyle protocols help shift the hormonal balance gently but powerfully.

Detox Routines

Detoxification facilitates efficient processing and elimination of excess estrogen to prevent reabsorption. Key mechanisms to enhance this process daily include:

Dry Brushing: Using a dry brush with stiff natural bristles brushing towards the heart before showering supports lymphatic drainage, exfoliates skin and reduces cellulite. Aim for 5-10 minutes daily.

Alternating Hydrotherapy: Alternate 1 minute hot and 30 second cold water cycles during your shower increases circulation and stimulates the lymphatic system to enhance drainage and detoxification.

Sauna Therapy: Portable saunas allow induced sweating to promote release and excretion of stored toxins and used hormones like estrogen. Combine with dry brushing before use and stay hydrated. Even 10 minutes a few times a week is extremely beneficial.

Oil Pulling: Swish 1 Tbsp organic cold pressed coconut or sesame oil in mouth for 10-20 minutes then spit out. Helps draws out toxins.

Skin Massage: Using a body oil or lotion 2-3 times a week, massage skin head to toe (towards lymph nodes) 10-15 minutes to stimulate drainage. Gua sha tools can enhance benefits.

Be sure to give your body plenty of fluids, electrolytes and minerals during detoxes especially if you experience any fatigue, headaches etc.

Stress and Lifestyle Reset

High stress directly triggers excess cortisol and estrogen production which overwhelms detox pathways. Press pause and practice self-care:

Daily Stress Relief Activities (10-20 min)

- Breathwork
- Guided meditations
- Journaling
- Walking in nature

Sleep Hygiene Tips

- Room darkening strategies
- Limit screen time before bed
- Melatonin and magnesium supplements if insomnia

Make Time For Joy!

- Connect with loved ones
- Practice a hobby

- Try easy wins like an Epsom salt bath

Deep restorative activities and pleasure allow your body to channel energy towards correcting underlying imbalances - a pivotal piece ignored in most health protocols!

Herbs and Supplement Recommendations

Herbal therapies and quality supplements provide concentrated phytonutrient support:

Hormone Balancing Formulations
Diindolylmethane (DIM), Vitex, Maca, Black Cohosh help metabolic pathways and promote equilibrium. Follow dosing guidelines.

Liver Support
Milk thistle, turmeric, glutathione recycling nutrients NAC and ALA enhance liver detoxification power.

Adaptogens Holy basil, ashwagandha and astragalus lower cortisol, protect adrenal glands and reduce inflammatory stress.

Whole Food Vitamins High quality multi-vitamins, activated B vitamins provide foundational micronutrient support missing from modern diets.

Work with your chosen health provider to curate targeted supplements addressing your hormonal symptoms and root causes. Timing of herbal doses can depend on cycle phase - track using provided symptom journals.

The above holistic protocols work synergistically with the dietary recommendations through the 28 days to facilitate deep healing shifts. Be easy with yourself during this process - progress over perfection!

Tracking Your Progress

Monitoring symptoms and progress empowers you to gauge what's working, customize protocols and stay motivated.

Use the following templates to track on a scale of 1-10:

Symptom Journal

Download printable copies to fill at the same time daily or use an app if easier.

- Bloating/swelling
- Breast tenderness
- Fatigue
- Migraines/headaches
- Sleep quality
- Mood - irritability, anxiety, low mood
- Clarity of thinking/brain fog
- Sex drive
- Any additional personal symptoms

Compare day-to-day as well as look for longer term weekly patterns. This helps identify potential hormonal cycle correlations and refine supplements.

Share your metrics with your functional medicine provider to inform treatment adjustments.

Follow-up Testing

Initial lab testing establishes your baseline to compare progress as metabolites and hormones fluctuate rapidly.

Re-test key markers after 2-3 months on the protocol:

- Estradiol
- Progesterone
- Testosterone
- DHEAS
- SHBG
- Fast blood glucose/insulin
- Inflammatory markers like hsCRP
- Micronutrient panel to check for deficiencies
- Stress hormones like cortisol variants to assess adrenal function

Beyond hormone and blood labs, consider repeat:

- DEXA scan for body composition changes
- Thermography screen for cellular inflammation
- Genetic panels to uncover methylation issues impacting detox
- Food sensitivity testing for potential elimination diet optimization

Analyzing trends in the above biomarkers indicates where your body needs additional support. Continue partnering with your functional health provider to interpret results in context and personalize follow-up protocols.

Celebrate Your Wins!

Don't forget to acknowledge and appreciate the positive shifts unfolding week-to-week even if gradual. Your dedication and resilience during this deep healing process is BADASS!

Potential Hurdles and Troubleshooting

As the body recalibrates, some temporary symptoms like headaches or fatigue can arise but subside quickly. Here's guidance for troubleshooting common scenarios:

Managing Detox Symptoms

Eliminating accumulated toxic estrogen and metabolizing stored forms to prep for excretion can be taxing temporarily. Support drainage pathways:

- Drink electrolyte liquids if tired or dizzy
- Allow extra rest if needed
- Try lymph drainage massage
- Reduce detox protocols if severe
- Communicate with your practitioner

Most symptoms resolve within 72 hours. Alleviating accumulated backlog gradually is smarter long-term than pushing aggressively.

Breaking Through Plateaus

If progress stalls, explore potential factors like:

Blood Sugar Imbalances

- Did you overdo high glycemic foods? Reel added sugars way back in
- Increase protein/healthy fat intake to stabilize blood sugar
- Take berberine, cinnamon or glucomannan before carb-heavy meals

Poor Liver Support

- Take a pause from supplements that burden liver like alpha lipoic acid
- Increase turmeric, milk thistle and liver loving whole foods

Hormonal Disruptors

- Identify and eliminate sneaky xenoestrogen sources
- Use only clean personal care and household products
- Check for hidden soy or hormones in packaged goods

Micronutrient Deficiency

- Rotate food groups to prevent developing deficiencies

- Incorporate a broad spectrum multi-vitamin
- Increase prebiotic fiber intake for microbial health

Inadequate Stress Relief

- Adrenal glands may need more targeted adaptogenic herbs
- Add relaxing rituals like breathwork, Epsom salt baths, enjoyable activities

Layering solutions that troubleshoot all potential weak links provides the reboot your body needs. Be patient, you've got this!

Chapter 3: Reducing Exposure to Estrogen-Like Compounds

Now that we have covered dietary and lifestyle interventions to facilitate hormone detoxification pathways in the body, this chapter focuses on reducing intake and exposure to external estrogen mimicking compounds.

As discussed earlier, these xenoestrogens or environmental estrogens from products, medications and environments burden the body contributing to overall excessive estrogenic activity. Minimizing contact can alleviate symptoms substantially.

We'll examine major sources of xenoestrogens and practical, actionable steps you can implement right away to avoid them.

Xenoestrogens in Food and Consumer Products

Plastics

Plastics contain hormone disrupting phthalates and bisphenol compounds like the infamous BPA that are omnipresent in food packaging, water bottles, plastic containers etc. Reheating and microwaving food in plastic ware makes leaching worse.

Solutions:

- Use glass, stainless steel or ceramic containers for storing and reheating food and liquids instead of plastic ware.

- Avoid canned foods and drinks lined with BPA in the coating.

- Use paper or reusable bags for storing and carrying items rather than plastic bags.

- Do not microwave food in plastic containers - transfer to glassware first.

Conventionally Raised Meat and Dairy

Commercially farmed livestock and dairy are routinely given synthetic hormones and antibiotics to accelerate growth which accumulate in tissues and milk. Opt for organic, grass-fed meat and dairy options to avoid ingesting these hormones and support ethical farming.

Solutions:

- Choose organic, grass-fed, hormone and antibiotic free meats as budget allows.

- Limit dairy intake to organic yogurt, butter and ghee minimally.

- For vegans, emphasize cleaner protein sources like organic lentils, beans and soy.

Pesticides and Herbicides

Growing research on glyphosate and atrazine reveals estrogenic effects negatively impacting fertility, menstruation, metabolism and triggering PCOS and fatigue.

Solutions:

- Buy certified organic produce, grains especially corn and soy where possible.
- Wash all produce thoroughly before eating.
- Grow own herbs and veggies at home if possible.
- Install water filters to minimize ingesting from tap water.

Parabens in Personal Care Products

This sneaky preservative mimics estrogen and is commonly found in makeup, shampoos, lotions and hair care products even listed as methylparaben, ethylparaben etc.

Solutions:

- Seek out clean, organic personal care brands without parabens.
- Use products certified by EWG's Skin Deep database to be low in toxins.
- DIY safe versions for cosmetics like lotions and hair masks using natural ingredients.

Food Dyes and Emulsifiers

Artificial food additives like dyes (Red No 40, Yellow No 6) and emulsifiers enable longer shelf life but are linked to hormone disruption and reproductive issues in studies.

Solutions:

- Check ingredient labels and avoid artificial dyes and emulsifiers like carrageenan and polysorbate 60/80 in foods.
- Consume more whole, natural foods - the less packaged and processed the better.
- Prepare homemade versions of sauces, salad dressings etc instead of buying.

Soy Products

While fermented organic soy in moderation provides benefits, heavily processed forms of soy like isolates, TVP and fake meats contain high phytoestrogens levels that outweigh the positives when consumed daily.

Solutions:

- Enjoy edamame, miso, tempeh and organic tofu sparingly.
- Avoid soy based meat replacements and protein powders with soy isolates.
- Choose alternate protein sources like sprouted legumes, eggs, hemp etc. instead.

Phytoestrogens from sources like flax seeds can also vary in effects based on gut health, microbiome makeup and estrogen levels. Hence moderating intake based on response is prudent.

Through an elimination diet removing inflammatory foods and reducing intake of the above xenoestrogens, you help ease the collective estrogen burden on the body.

Estrogen Promoters in Medications and Cosmetics

Beyond directly ingesting and absorbing these synthetic hormones, many routinely prescribed drugs and beauty products also indirectly promote higher circulating estrogen levels or inhibit detox pathways.

Oral Contraceptives

The birth control pill with formulations of synthetic estrogen and progestin prevents ovulation but also increases sex hormone binding globulin levels. This binds up free testosterone, lowering the ratio of progesterone to estrogen.

Long term pill use is also linked to depleted nutrient reserves involved in detox pathways worsening symptoms.

Solutions:

- Discuss alternate non hormonal birth control options with your doctor.
- Address potential underlying issues like PCOS, endometriosis or amenorrhea driving use rather than just masking symptoms.
- Replenish depleted micronutrient reserves if stopping.

Hormone Replacement Therapy

Intended to relieve menopausal symptoms, traditional HRT with equine or synthetic estrogen alone disrupts natural rhythms in the body worsening fatigue, clotting etc. Effects can persist years after stopping.

Solutions:

- Explore bioidentical hormone therapy customized to your needs.
- Try safer herbal supplements before resorting to HRT.
- Make comprehensive diet and lifestyle upgrades specific to perimenopause.

Antidepressant Medications

Drugs like SSRIs for depression, anxiety and OCD have been found to stimulate higher levels of estrogen production along with lower testosterone. This is believed to drive issues like weight gain, insomnia and headaches as side effects.

Solutions:

- Discuss psychological counseling, mind-body techniques to wean off medication under medical guidance.
- Actively make lifestyle upgrades lowering inflammation and supporting neurotransmitter balance through dietary amino acids, movement, stress reduction techniques etc. instead of relying solely on medication.

Topical Creams

Counterintuitively, hydrocortisone cream applied topically can increase estrogen absorption and lower progesterone levels. So can any emulsions that compromise skin barrier integrity long term. Evaluate if common topical prescriptions are worsening hormonal issues.

Solutions:

- Avoid repetitive application of topical steroids and lotions without letting skin recover, unless absolutely medically necessary.

- Use safer alternatives like calendula salves to support skin healing.

- Identify and eliminate triggers causing dermatitis flare ups, through allergy testing if required.

Similarly some chemical based cosmetic products and hair lotions contain placental extracts and estrogens that boost systemic levels. Pay attention if symptoms appear correlated to when using specific beauty products.

The goal here is not to vilify all modern medicine or cosmetics but rather equip you to make informed decisions through deeper questioning. Sometimes medication is indispensable - so work with your doctors to balance need with unwanted impacts.

Now that we have covered common environmental and pharmaceutical sources of estrogen promotion and interference with breakdown, let's explore nourishing the liver's detox capabilities.

Supporting Detox Pathways

The liver plays over 500 roles within the body! Two key aspects in relation to estrogen dominance involve:

1. Producing binding proteins that transport key hormones like estrogen safely.

2. Detoxifying and breaking down excess hormones into inactive metabolites.

Enhancing these liver detoxification systems can have an instrumental effect on alleviating symptoms driven by hormone buildup and toxicity.

The liver processes external toxins and old hormones in 2 phases:

Phase 1: Enzymes known as the cytochrome P450 family oxidize molecules making them more water soluble for excretion using nutrients like B vitamins, vitamin C, zinc and magnesium.

Phase 2: Additional enzymatic reactions convert compounds into safe excretable forms by processes like methylation requiring nutrients such as glycine, sulfur, potassium etc.

Fine tuning intake of these essential macro and micronutrients through real food nourishes the liver machinery handling hormone regulation and turnover. Let's explore additional avenues to enhance detox mechanisms.

Herbal Support

Certain botanicals enhance health at a cellular level and aid the liver's cleansing processes. Some prime examples validated by research include:

Milk Thistle: Silymarin flavonoids within milk thistle protect liver tissue from incoming toxins while increasing production of glutathione - the master antioxidant and detoxifier. Enhances both Phase 1 and 2 enzyme action aiding steroid hormone metabolism.

Turmeric: Curcumin compounds in turmeric reduce fat buildup in liver while enhancing Phase 2 pathways involved in estrogen breakdown and clearance. Helps metabolize excess estrogens circulating back from the intestines further lowering burden.

Schisandra: This adaptogenic herb increases levels of the key antioxidant glutathione along with liver enzymes that inactivate and clear high estrogen loads. Also protects and repairs liver damage enabling better hormone processing.

Artichoke Extract: Potent antioxidant and bile stimulant promoting optimal fat digestion and prevention of estrogen reabsorption during enterohepatic circulation for higher net excretion. Contains liver regenerative compounds.

Herbal Bitters: Bitter herbs like dandelion, milk thistle, goldenseal etc. stimulate digestive secretions improving gut motility and liver function. Preventing estrogen reuptake further reduces recirculating loads.

Ginseng: Used traditionally to relieve menstrual and menopausal discomfort, ginseng improves estrogen detox via supporting liver function and glandular system recovery. Also aids stress adaptation reducing cortisol loads.

Dosing on effective amounts guided by your functional medicine practitioner helps leverage synergistic actions of herbs above with minimal side effects.

Nutritional Compounds

Vitamins like B12, B6, folate and trace minerals like zinc are involved as cofactors in the liver detox pathways facilitating removal of used hormones from the body. Deficiencies can severely stall mechanisms increasing toxicity.

Solutions:

- Test for and correct any nutritional deficiencies blocking detox pathways through whole food sources first before extensive supplementation.

- Reduce alcohol and medications depleting stores.

- Stabilize digestion using HCL, enzymes and probiotics if gut dysfunction is malabsorbing nutrients.

The liver also requires antioxidants to quench inflammatory and oxidative damage from toxin exposure while regenerating tissue. Key antioxidant rich foods include:

Glutathione foods: Asparagus, avocado, spinach, squash, grapefruit etc.

SOD foods: Beets, purple sweet potatoes leafy greens, spirulina, wheatgrass

Catalase foods: Sweet potatoes, spinach and cruciferous vegetables

Feeding your body's innate detoxification potential by reducing intake of xenohormones while optimizing liver flow is pivotal. Now let's cover additional detox practices and pathways.

Enhancing Gastrointestinal Motility and Microbiome Balance

The small intestine and colon play an important role in managing estrogen levels through:

1. Binding and excreting excess estrogens so less is reabsorbed.

2. Converting less potent estrogens like estrone into protective metabolites before they recirculate enterohepatically.

Gut flow and transit time impact how effectively estrogen is eliminated preventing rising exposure. Slow motility gives more time for reuptake and dysbiosis alters detoxification capacity of intestinal flora.

Solutions:

- Test and treat underlying causes of extra-intestinal symptoms like small intestinal bacterial overgrowth (SIBO) if suspected which hamper transit.

- Ensure 30-40 grams fiber daily from fruits, vegetables and nuts keeping bowels regular.

- Stay well hydrated with 8+ glasses filtered water to support detox mechanisms and flush waste.

- Practice regular movement – exercise, walking, Pilates etc that gently stimulate circulation and peristalsis furthering elimination.

Certain amino acids like glycine and glutamine along with minerals like magnesium serve as gut restore and protect agents reducing inflammation enabling waste clearance. Bone broth delivers easily absorbed forms making it a nourishing traditional food for healing leaky, inflamed or slowed guts.

Probiotics to Modulate Estrogen Metabolism

Healthy gut flora contains certain beneficial bacteria that break down and excrete surplus estrogen helping prevent buildup and enterohepatic recirculation through processes like:

- **Deconjugating Estrogens:** Intestinal bacteria cleave apart used estrogens from carrier compounds pumping them back into circulation prolonging toxicity. Specific probiotics assist this allowing quicker elimination.

- **Estrogen Metabolism:** Certain strains metabolize potent estrogens like estradiol converting them into weaker estriol and estrone preventing reabsorption intensity while also inhibiting enzymes that synthesize estrogens internally.

In this light, enhancing the colonies of health-promoting flora through frequent probiotic and fermented food intake becomes particularly useful when addressing high estrogen issues.

Liver - Gut Axis

This interlinked axis is crucial to balance since poor liver function directly affects gut lining integrity and vice versa in a perpetual cycle.

Fixing one without addressing the other typically leads to relapse. Key pathways impacted include:

- Bile flow and constituents – impaired with fatty liver disease leads to poor fat digestion, bacterial overgrowth from bile acid changes and greater estrogen reabsorption.

- Microbiome disruption from drugs, alcohol etc produce toxic metabolites that burden the liver stalling healthy hormone breakdown.

Hence a dual pronged focus on restoring microbial balance and liver flow simultaneously has profound expanding benefits.

In summary, reducing intake of endocrine disrupting compounds, supporting liver pathways breaking down hormones while optimizing waste elimination capacity together lower total estrogen load substantially easing related symptoms and future disease risks.

Chapter 4: Supporting Estrogen Metabolism and Elimination

In this chapter, we will dig deeper into key nutrients, herbs and pathways directly involved in healthy estrogen metabolism.

Optimizing these processes facilitates breakdown and swift elimination preventing used estrogens from recirculating inappropriately.

We will also cover testing related biomarkers providing insight on specific areas of dysfunction that could be stalling your hormone detox.

Nutrients Supporting Estrogen Detoxification

Let's begin with key vitamins, minerals and antioxidants that serve as cofactors supporting the liver's near 500 functions including managing estrogen levels.

B Vitamins

The entire B-complex group of vitamins participates in estrogen breakdown, building hormones and neurotransmitters, detox reactions etc. Deficiencies severely stall these interlinked pathways.

Solutions:

Test levels especially B12, folate, B6 and address any shortfalls with food sources first before extensive supplementation under guidance.

B12: Boost intake via grass-fed meats, seafood, eggs and nut milks. Supports methylation.

B6: Up vitamin B6 levels consuming poultry, potato skins, pistachios. Catalyzes toxicity processing.

Folate rich: Spinach, beef liver, black eyed peas supply folate aiding hormone balance.

B-Complex: Take an activated B-complex supplement with adequate B12, methylated folate etc. proportionate to needs upon testing.

Magnesium

One of the most common nutritional inadequacies, low magnesium impedes hundreds of reactions like blood sugar regulation, detox enzyme function, inflammation control etc. worsening hormone issues.

Up to 80% of women do not meet RDA levels for this mineral also lost through stress, alcohol and medications.

Solutions:

Test magnesium in RBC rather than serum which can mask tissue depletion.

Consume more: Leafy greens, pumpkin seeds, cocoa, avocado, salmon and Epsom salt baths boost reserves.

Supplement forms like glycinate, malate, citrate etc. with medical guidance on ideal elemental dosage based on deficiency.

Zinc

This trace mineral plays extensive roles ranging from immunity to healthy skin, eyes, hormones etc. Deficiencies directly affect estrogen pathway enzymes and metabolism.

Alcohol consumption, insulin resistance and malnutrition hamper absorption rates leading to complications.

Solutions:

- **Test for zinc adequacy** – ideal level is above 100 ng/ml range.
- Up bioavailable food sources such as oysters, eggs, pumpkin seeds and grass-fed beef.
- Limit copper exposure from low zinc.
- Check for H.pylori overgrowth if levels remain persistently low despite diet changes.
- **Supplement:** Typical dosage around 25-50 mg elemental zinc picolinate, glycinate or citrate forms.

Vitamin D

- Low vitamin D is strongly correlated with menstrual irregularities, estrogen dominant symptoms etc. Raise levels testing and optimizing accordingly.
- **Solutions**: Get more safe sun exposure. Include egg yolks, sardines, liver and mushrooms.
- **Supplement:** Take Vitamin D3 + K2 forms based on retesting for more sustainable improvements long term.

Vitamin C

Potent anti-inflammatory and antioxidant protecting liver tissues from incoming toxins and waste products. Vitamin C recycles other antioxidants like vitamin E and glutathione furthering their protective effects against excess estrogen issues.

Solutions:

- **Test Vitamin C levels** – optimal above 45 μmol/L with additional buffer quantity desired.

- Citrus fruits, bell peppers, strawberries and broccoli boost dietary vitamin C intake.

- **Supplement** C complex for higher antioxidant support as needed.

Selenium

Works closely with vitamin E, glutathione and vitamin C within liver pathways neutralizing free radicals and harmful estrogen metabolites preventing cellular damage and recirculation.

Deficiency correlates strongly with issues like hypothyroidism and autoimmunity that exacerbate estrogen dominance.

Solutions:

- **Test levels:** Optimally 100-130 ng/ml range.

- Brazil nuts, sardines, eggs, chicken breast and spinach increase bioavailable selenium.

- Take 200 mcg methylated selenium capsules with mixed tocopherols based on testing guidance.

Through correcting common nutritional inadequacies, you better support the body's inbuilt capacity for breaking down and eliminating surplus estrogens via the liver pathway.

Now let's discuss key botanicals and plant compounds facilitating this.

Botanicals Supporting Healthy Estrogen Metabolism

Certain adaptogenic herbs directly aid liver enzymes, promote gut integrity for higher net estrogen excretion, and reduce inflammatory damage preventing estrogen recirculation.

The gentle holistic effects make these botanicals ideal to boost the body's hormone balancing efforts. Let's cover some prime plant allies:

Milk Thistle

The silymarin complex within milk thistle protects liver cell health from incoming hormone metabolites and toxins.

It increases production of glutathione – the master cellular detoxifier and enhances liver regeneration.

By supporting Phase I and Phase II detox action, it specifically facilitates dismantling used estrogens for complete clearance out of the body.

Dosage for hormone balance: **150-300 mg silymarin complex with phosphatidylcholine 2-3x daily.**

Ginger

Ginger contains antioxidant gingerols that alleviate inflammatory damage, improve gut motility preventing reabsorption of estrogens and modulate estrogen receptor pathways reducing symptoms.

It further stimulates liver detoxification enzymes that process and break down excess circulating estrogen loads for efficient elimination.

Dosage for hormone balance: **1000 – 2000 mg fresh ginger or ginger extract daily**

Turmeric

The bioactive curcumin within turmeric reduces inflammatory damage and learns fatty liver disease preventing toxin buildup.

It is shown to positively modulate enzymes like GST and GAPDH involved in the liver's Phase II detox of estrogens making their clearance more effective.

Turmeric also mitigates high circulating estrogen from re-entering the enterohepatic circulation further lowering recirculating burden.

Dosage for hormone balance: **500 mg to 1000 mg turmeric curcumin supplements daily**

Grapefruit Seed Extract

Contains antioxidant compounds that stimulate cleansing of liver detoxification pathways easing the burden of estrogen and other used hormones waiting to be processed and excreted.

Also beneficial for promoting healthy gut flora balance aiding elimination. Dosage: **150 to 300 mg grapefruit seed extract capsules daily.**

Green Tea Extract

Abundant EGCG catechins make green tea a powerful antioxidant protecting liver tissue from incoming toxin induced damage.

It is also shown to upregulate production of crucial liver enzymes and glutathione levels facilitating liver's breakdown of estrogen, xenoestrogens, medications etc.

Dosage: **250 to 500 mg green tea extract capsules per day.**

When combined synergistically, herbs and botanicals above gently provide liver support, improve estrogen metabolism enzymes, reduce intermediates while assisting detox mechanisms easing clearance and related symptoms.

Testing Related Biomarkers to Assess Detox Dysfunction

Alongside adding vitamins, minerals and herbs, identifying potential issues interfering with optimal estrogen breakdown can further customize care.

Let's cover key associated labs and functional markers to test.

Liver Function Panel

At the very minimum, get annual checks on common markers indicating how well your liver is metabolizing hormones and toxins:

ALT and AST: Elevated levels indicate liver cell damage that impairs detox capability.

Alkaline Phosphatase: Higher amounts point to inhibited bile flow necessary to prevent reuptake of estrogens.

Bilirubin: Increased or very low bilirubin reflects liver stagnancy issues and needs further evaluation.

Albumin: Chronically low albumin indicates liver inability to synthesize compounds essential for hormone transport and detox.

Verify any aberrations by further testing:

Liver Imaging

Get imaging like ultrasound, MRI or CT scan to check for fatty liver disease. Excess liver fat disrupts hormone breakdown pathways substantially.

Toxic Load Markers

Elevated heavy metals, biotoxins (mold), plastic compounds (phthalates) etc. overwhelm liver machinery and directly alter hormone synthesis and breakdown.

Comprehensive tests like toxicant screen panels and mycotoxin assays help gauge total load.

Phase I and Phase II Detox Function

Laboratory urine testing analyzes use of challenge agents like caffeine to check sufficiency of key liver P450 detox enzymes.

Low clearance of indicators like paraxanthine reflects issues in efficiently cycling estrogen out.

Consider genetic testing analyzing Single Nucleotide Polymorphisms affecting liver health as well guiding custom support needs.

Now that you understand the intricate dance between liver detox pathways and healthy estrogen breakdown, let's cover the pivotal role nutrition plays in rebalancing this key system.

Chapter 5: The Critical Roles of Nutrition and Diet

Nutrition plays a pivotal yet commonly overlooked role when it comes to balancing hormones and easing unpleasant symptoms associated with estrogen dominance.

The food we eat provides the raw materials to build and regulate every tissue, gland and metabolic pathway within our body. Optimizing intake of nutrients that facilitate healthy estrogen metabolism while avoiding dietary components that hinder it can create radical positive shifts.

This chapter details evidence-based guidance on therapeutic foods, nutrients and compounds to emphasize as well as ones to limit or avoid to reclaim hormonal harmony through the dietary dimension.

Estrogen Balancing Foods to Focus On

Prioritizing anti-inflammatory, antioxidant rich, fiber containing real foods in their whole forms while ensuring adequate healthy fats, plant/animal protein and micronutrients provides immense healing benefits.

Anti-Inflammatory Foods

Systemic inflammation drives estrogen dominance by impairing liver detoxification, disrupting digestion, causing obesity and directly altering hormonal pathways.

Choosing foods recognized to reduce inflammatory cytokines and increase protective metabolites helps relieve related symptoms. These include:

Colorful Fruits and Vegetables: The vibrant polyphenols within berries, pomegranates, purple grapes and compounds in leafy greens, cruciferous vegetables, onions and mushrooms possess robust anti-inflammatory effects protecting estrogen sensitive tissues.

Herbs and Spices: Turmeric, ginger, garlic, cumin, cinnamon, oregano contain potent plant bioactives that reduce inflammatory COX/LOX enzymes and histamine secretion easing headaches, breast and abdominal discomfort, fluid retention.

Fatty Fish: Omega-3s in salmon, mackerel, sardines exert anti-inflammatory action. Can help lower fibrotic breast tissue density and menstrual pain. Choose low mercury wild caught varieties.

Nuts and Seeds: Anti-oxidant reserves within almonds, walnuts, flax, pumpkin and chia seeds reduce inflammatory triggers caused by poor diet, obesity and stress imbalance. Contain healthy fats and fiber further aiding hormone regulation.

Green Tea/Rooibos Tea: Catechins within quality green tea are renowned inflammation fighters. Rooibos is an herb rich in liver protective antioxidants, minerals that aid estrogen breakdown.

Extra Virgin Olive Oil: Powerful plant compounds called oleocanthal give olive oil unique COX enzyme inhibitory potential easing aches, discomfort, oxidative and inflammatory drivers of high estrogen load.

Fermented Foods: Naturally probiotic foods like kefir, kimchi, pickles, sauerkraut contain organic acids and living cultures that reduce inflammatory cytokines, prostaglandins and histamine.

Antioxidant-Rich Foods

Oxidative damage from poor nutrition, toxicity accumulation and high stress burdens hormone regulatory systems and the liver necessitating antioxidant-rich nutrients. Some prime sources include:

Dark leafy Greens: Spinach, kale and microgreens highest in detox enzymes glutathione, SOD, catalase which quench free radicals stalled estrogen metabolism produces.

Brightly Colored Produce: Bioflavonoids within berries neutralize excess estrogen and support pathway integrity. Lycopene in tomatoes and carotenoids in carrots, sweet potatoes act as antioxidants.

Sprouted Seeds/Legumes: Sprouting dramatically increases antioxidant capacity and nutrient density within beans, seeds and grains through activating potent enzymes that aid liver and hormone health. Particularly rich in B-vitamins and zinc involved in pathways of estrogen and toxin elimination.

Herbs and Spices: Turmeric, cinnamon, oregano, cilantro, basil contain a spectrum of antioxidant polyphenols which restore optimal tissue function and antioxidant reserves.

Cacao: Raw cacao uniquely contains dense quantities of antioxidants that protect cell membranes from harm, reduce inflammation and damage to glandular tissues caused by environmental toxins and metabolic waste accumulation. Enhances detox enzymes.

Wild-Caught Fish: Omega-3 fats within lower mercury containing wild salmon, mackerel and sardines enhance antioxidative protection through direct radical scavenging action and inflammatory modulation preventing estrogen overload caused tissue damage and fibroids.

Fiber-Rich Foods

Adequate daily fiber is critical for binding and eliminating excess circulating estrogen from the body preventing reabsorption and enterohepatic recirculation back into tissues when gut flow is compromised.

Some of the best high fiber food sources encompass:

Leafy Greens: Dark leafy greens like spinach, swiss chard and cruciferous vegetables have very high fiber levels aiding elimination of waste estrogen metabolites. Also deliver antioxidant protection.

Berries: Raspberries and blackberries help post-menopausal weight loss while blueberries enhance cardiovascular benefits through improving cholesterol efflux - all via fiber rich mechanisms beneficial in estrogen dominance reversal.

Root Vegetables: Dense in soluble and insoluble fiber fractions, beets, sweet potatoes and yams help enhance digestive elimination preventing constipation while feeding gut flora. Fiber lowers high estrogen reabsorption directly and indirectly by reducing obesity driving excess aromatase enzyme activity and circulating estrogen levels in the first place.

Chia Seeds: Just 1-2 tbsp delivers nearly 10 grams of high viscous fiber proven to modulate hormone levels, improve metabolic markers and manage healthy body weight - powerful mechanisms to counter estrogen promoter paths. The omega-3s within further drive anti-inflammatory action.

Oats and Barley: Excellent sources of beta-glucan fiber beneficial for cardiovascular health, bowel regularity and lowering cholesterol. Assists weight loss in estrogen dominant populations reducing excess aromatization of testosterone to high estrogen loads. Can reduce breast density and symptoms.

Wheat Bran: The outer husk fraction contains highest fiber fractions to enhance transit supporting liver bile flow and toxin elimination through feces instead of reuptake. Useful addition but avoid wheat/gluten if sensitive.

Beans: Fiber rich, nutrient dense kidney beans, chickpeas, black beans and lentils further aid healthy estrogen detox through mineral support of pathways while being plant-based protein sources that correct tissue amino acid needs without promoting intake of commercial meat factory farmed hormones.

Psyllium Husk: Pure powder from the Plantago ovata shrub is very high in soluble and insoluble fiber with the ability to improve liver function, detoxification enzyme activity, bile flow etc by optimizing gastrointestinal motility and waste elimination preventing toxin overload.

Micronutrient and Phytonutrient-Rich Foods

Key vitamins, minerals and protective plant compounds are required to run the intricate orchestra of enzymes, cofactors, proteins and pathways regulating healthy estrogen metabolism.

Deficiencies or inadequacies in these nutrient reserves distort function enabling high or unopposed estrogen to exert dominant symptoms. Emphasizing foods containing these aids hormone balance:

B-Vitamins (Thiamine, Riboflavin, Niacin, Pantothenic Acid): Essential for liver Phase 1 detox generating enzymes and processes breaking down potent estrogens for elimination. Also needed for building progesterone counter-balancing estrogens.

Magnesium: Critical mineral involved in over 300 enzyme processes including nutrients activating pathways to metabolize and excrete excess estrogens. Needed for DNA and oxidative repair from toxicity burdens.

Zinc: Both zinc and B6 play vital roles in liver CYP enzymes governing estrogen breakdown. Also protects cell membranes from environmental toxin damage enabling proper hormone cell receptor function preventing overload.

Calcium D-Glucarate: Cruciferous contain this phytonutrient that aids liver detox through glucuronidation leading to urinary estrogen excretion lowering reuptake. Enhances kidney elimination.

Green Tea Catechins: The unique catechins from unprocessed quality green tea aid liver detoxification, provide antioxidant protection, reduce breast cancer proliferation markers and lower serum estrogen levels significantly through a multitude of protective actions.

Resveratrol (Grapes): This anti-aging antioxidant in grape skins, peanuts and fruits demonstrate selective estrogen modulator (SERM) like activity enhancing protective estrogen metabolism via the healthier CYP1A1 pathway reducing DNA damage and cancer risks from potent estrogens.

Allium Family: Organosulfur compounds within cruciferous vegetables, onions and garlic up-regulate liver detoxifying enzymes, support methylation pathways and protect DNA while suppressing generation of excess estrogens - highly protective allium phytochemicals.

Brassica Family: Alongside fiber and antioxidants, compounds like indole-3 carbinol and sulforaphane in cruciferous vegetables aid healthier Phase 1 CYP enzyme activity and the critical Phase 2 liver detoxifying step of glucuronidation facilitating elimination of hazardous estrogen metabolites and toxins.

Healthy Fats and Oils

While excess body fat triggers substantially greater estrogen production through the enzyme aromatase, adequate anti-inflammatory fats provide tissue protection against hormone disruption, modulation of eicosanoid hormone synthesis and lowering high levels through multiple channels. Beneficial fats and oils encompass:

Extra Virgin Olive Oil: Powerful anti-inflammatory oleic acid lowers inflammatory prostaglandin E2 promoting healthy estrogen balance easing sore breasts, bloating etc. Enhanced fat metabolism lowers obesity.

Omega-3 Fats: Alpha linolenic acid, EPA and DHA abundant in fatty fish, chia, flax and walnuts competitively inhibit inflammatory omega-6 ARA pathways reducing estrogen driven breast and uterine hyperplasia. Improve mood, pain and detox potential.

Coconut oil: Contains unique antifungal lauric acid and caprylic acid useful against candida overgrowth worsening estrogen dominance. Provides quick energy and supports thyroid hormone movement lowering risks of estrogen related autoimmune disease.

Ghee and Butter: Healthy saturated fats enhance cell membrane fluidity aiding hormone receptor function and signalling preventing issues like insulin resistance furthering fat driven excess estrogen. Short and medium chain fats support metabolism and detox.

Avocados: Anti-inflammatory monounsaturated fatty acids protect mood and cardiovascular health while the glutathione content counters liver toxicity enabling better estrogen breakdown. Provides antioxidant carotenoids and minerals activating pathways.

Additionally, adequate protein intake through ethical animal source or plant-based choices provides amino acid precursors supporting optimal community signaling and function while preventing the tendency towards stress and sugar craving blood sugar imbalances disrupting endocrine pathways.

Foods and Substances That Worsen Estrogen Dominance

Now that we have covered therapeutic foods to emphasize, let's examine common dietary compounds that can directly or indirectly raise estrogen activity and worsen related symptoms.

The goal is not extreme prohibition but rather reducing intake of these judiciously through conscious moderation and swapping healthier alternatives to provide the body optimal nutrition support.

Alcohol: Enhances conversion of androgens like testosterone into estrogens worsening imbalance. Strains detox organs like liver further preventing efficient estrogen breakdown.

Aggravates inflammation and gut permeability allowing greater reabsorption.

Caffeine: Excess intake overactivates stress pathways like cortisol secretion which indirectly negatively affects female hormonal balance through HPA axis suppression, adrenal strain, insulin resistance and obesity.

Processed Carbohydrates and Sugars: Drive cellular insulin resistance promoting inflation, belly weight gain and elevated aromatase enzyme activity converting androgens into estrogen exacerbating symptoms through fat driven surplus production overloading an already strained system.

Trans Fats and Vegetable Oils: Pro-inflammatory, gut irritating compounds that provide no nutritional benefit while accumulating as cellular toxicity creating free radical damage to hormone receptive tissues. Avoid completely through mindful label reading.

Conventional Dairy and Meat: Commercial cattle milk and beef contain synthetic steroid hormones and pesticide residues that accumulate with patents already struggling to clear their own endogenous excess estrogen load owing to compromised detox capabilities. Chose organic.

Unfermented Soy Products: Over-consumption of unfermented soy transfers unhealthy levels of phytoestrogens into the body further worsening surplus mimicking activities through receptor site competition and interference with protein synthesis of endogenous sex hormones. Stick to tempeh.

Gluten: Intolerance is common in women with menstrual cycle or fertility issues correlating to cross-reactivity and inflammation that potentiates problems of hormone dysregulation. Eliminate or confirm sensitivity through antibody testing if suspecting a role.

Microwaved Food in Plastics: Heating food causes plasticizers and phthalates like BPA to leach into meals introducing endocrine disrupting pseudo-estrogens that overwhelm clearance systems.

Leftover Parabens from Body Products: Parabens used widely as preservatives in cosmetics, skin creams and hair products are chemically similar in structure to estrogens and can exert pseudo-hormonal activity when accumulated in tissue over years of repeat usage as is common.

Through a focused elimination diet and food sensitivity testing, mindfully avoiding common triggers provides immense healing benefit rebalancing hormonal health and relieving associated discomforts.

Supporting Estrogen Breakdown Through Diet

Now that we have covered specific balancing and avoidant foods, let's consolidate evidence-based diet and lifestyle measures facilitating healthy estrogen metabolism:

Lower Body Fat Percentage: Reducing excess adipose tissue directly lowers the conversion of adrenal androgens like DHEA-s into potent estrogens via the aromatase enzyme densely concentrated in fat cells. Even a modest 8-10% loss significantly alleviates high estrogen.

Increase Cruciferous Intake: Vegetable family vastly documented to improve protective estrogen breakdown route via glucuronidation, reduce circulating levels of biologically active estrogens and enhance excretion potential - highly researched brassica benefits.

Ensure Nutritional Sufficiency: Many vitamins and minerals act as necessary co-factors and precursors in the elaborate enzyme systems responsible for estrogen synthesis, transport, receptor binding and metabolism. Assess and correct any critical deficiencies which may be stalling your progress.

Healthy Bowel Function: Improving gastrointestinal motility enhances clearance preventing reuptake and enterohepatic recirculation of estrogen. Adequate daily fiber with prebiotic veggies feeds gut flora producing beneficial compounds aiding liver detoxification.

Stress and Inflammatory Control: Mastering daily stressors through sufficient sleep, relaxation practices, mind-body therapies etc. reduces cortisol and inflammatory drivers of impaired detox function which indirectly exacerbate issues of estrogen overload and imbalance manifestation.

Adaptogenic Botanicals: Certain anti-stress and liver supporting herbs like milk thistle, turmeric, schizandra etc. accelerate recovery pathways correcting exhaustion of glandular organs like thyroid and adrenals which closely interact with female hormones governing optimal balance through cascading communication networks. Dose as appropriate.

Assess for Endocrine Disruptors: Environmental pseudo-estrogens add to issues so investigating exposure through hydration sources, foods stored or heated in plastic, parabens and skin product ingredients list etc. allows you to pinpoint and reduce contributory xenobiotic drivers comprising clearance.

Following these guidelines with consistency supports the body's innate drive towards equilibrium as hormones work in tightly choreographed rhythms easy to distort and require holisticReset for restoration. Progress may seem slow but small positive momentum aggregates expanding benefits.

Chapter 6: Beyond the 28 Days - Strategies for Hormonal Balance

Congrats on making it through the intensive 28-day intervention! By this point, you must have witnessed noticeable improvements, and likely been able to discontinue or minimize medications related to common symptoms of estrogen dominance.

Key first steps also involved addressing potential nutritional deficiencies, hidden food triggers, environmental toxins while establishing sustainable healthy lifestyle routines focused on restorative whole foods, stress resilience practices, movement and sleep.

But the journey does not stop here - the real integration actually begins now for the weeks and months beyond as you learn to consolidate and personalize positive changes attained for long lasting relief and vibrancy.

In this closing chapter, we'll discuss:

1. Individualizing The Diet and Lifestyle Plan
2. Ongoing Testing and Assessment
3. Supplements for Maintenance
4. Strategic Detoxification
5. Working with Your Doctor
6. Troubleshooting Challenges

7. Transitioning to Maintenance Phase

Equipped with the comprehensive understanding of underlying drivers, symptoms and interventions to improve estrogen detox developed through earlier chapters, you are now ready to integrate the fundamentals into customized protocols tweaked to fit your unique lifestyle, priorities, biochemical individuality for optimal hormonal equilibrium.

Customizing the Diet and Lifestyle Protocol

While research indicates several universal dietary and lifestyle measures like increasing cruciferous vegetables, lowering sugar intake, getting micronutrients etc. relieve hormone imbalance for most; individual variances in case histories, genetic SNPs, gut microbiome composition, metabolism etc. mean personalization dramatically amplifies therapeutic results for lasting success.

Here are key aspects to evaluate and modify:

Rotate Out New Anti-Inflammatory Foods

Keep introducing novel anti-inflammatory real foods not consumed before into daily meals for gut microbiome and palate variation while assessing impact on energy, skin, mood and cycle tracking symptoms.

Great additions include eating the rainbow with purple/red berries, green veggies, orange winter squash, integrating interesting herbs/spices like turmeric, oregano, eliminating suspect nightshades like tomatoes if sensitivity is suspected.

Keep a Food and Symptom Diary

Ongoing logging of all foods consumed including ounces, minutes of exercise, supplements taken and rating energy, mood, bowel movements, focus etc. daily enables you to correlate inputs to quality of results.

This helps pinpoint contributors or detractors of progress for appropriate inclusion and reduction. Apps and bullet journal templates help tracking easy.

Time Intermittent Fasting and Detox Days

Scheduling 16-48 hour fasts before, during and after your cycle strategically enhances cellular cleanup processes through autophagy, allows digestive rest while reducing inflammatory immune flare ups worsening symptoms.

Herbal teas, electrolytes and bone broth aid compliance over pure water fasts only. Similarly occasional raw juice or smoothie detox days give the digestive tract reprieve.

Emphasize Circadian Living

Optimizing circadian cues through consistent bed-times, melatonin support, blue light blocking, scheduled meal times and exercise trains hormones like cortisol for lower output allowing restorative sleep, growth hormone release and reduced insulin resistance crucial for metabolic and reproductive health.

Stress Relief Practices

Reading, meditating, forest bathing, swimming, adaptogenic herbs - find those routines evoking relaxation response supplying parasympathetic nervous system activation enabling recovery from chronic stress stimulus which indirectly worsens hormonal pathways through elevated cortisol, blood sugar spikes, obesity, thyroid burnout, neurotransmitter dysregulation, gut inflammation and thus poor cycling.

Minimize Endocrine Disruptors

Filtering water, buying clean skin/hair care products, prioritizing glass over plastics may seem small measures but reduce xeno-estrogen and heavy metal buildup that tax clearance mechanisms distorting function over months and years - hence vital for sensitive individuals to reduce allostatic load.

Through daily and weekly check-ins assessing what lifestyle tweaks make you feel consistently vibrant and ease worrisome symptoms versus what detracts from progress, the self discovery process allows attaining long term balance.

Follow Up Testing and Medical Assessment

While you may feel significantly better after the 28 days owing to reduced inflammation, improved diet, detox and supplements, objective testing provides pivotal validation and additional customization insight. Hence follow up lab testing helps assess:

1. Hormone Level Changes

Getting retested levels of key sex hormones like estradiol, progesterone, DHEA-S, SHBG etc. in weeks or months after the intensive phase lets you quantify objective improvements in values, ratios and understand any persisting imbalances or new developments for precision correction.

2. Detox and Metabolic Biomarkers

Testing oxidative stress, liver enzymes, inflammatory cytokines, fasting insulin etc. paints an accurate picture of to what degree systemic burden has lowered along with metabolic parameters indicating if continuing symptoms may be downstream effects of yet unchecked dysfunctions requiring specialized support.

3. Nutritional and Microbiome Markers

Checking follow up vitamin D, B12, ferritin, zinc etc. identifies any corrected or lingering deficiencies causing symptoms like hair fall or fatigue while microbiome analysis via stool tests assess if gut flora changes enhanced beneficial compounds, diversity and reduced opportunistic organisms maintaining progress.

Follow up testing helps make definitive correlations between a dietary addition you made like increased phytoestrogen foods or probiotic drinks taken and actual measurable improvements in medical metrics – enabling you to independently validate and solidify positive lifestyle programs for lasting success.

Supplements for Ongoing Support

Here are some key supplement categories alongside optimal doses for maintenance:

Probiotics - 20-50 billion units daily from multi-strain, shelf-stable formulas containing strains like Lactobacillus helveticus which break down hormone metabolites. Can rotate through different price points for diversity.

Adaptogens - Rhodiola, Ashwagandha, Holy Basil standardized extracts up to 500-1000mg daily in cycles support stress adaptation, cortisol regulation benefitting thyroid-adrenal crosstalk, waistline and blood sugar management indirectly optimizing hormonal pathways.

Calcium d-Glucarate - 200-500mg daily supplies this liver supporting nutrient which enhances binding and elimination of used estrogens via stools instead of reabsorption and recirculation.

DIM + Broccoli Supplements - Pairing estrogen metabolite balancing DIM with I3C, sulforaphane containing broccoli powder/extract supplements ensures optimal detox pathways and cellular equilibrium are maintained after intensive phase corrections.

Omega 3s - 1000-2000mg daily through triglyceride form omega-3s derived from fish oil and algal sources ensures you maintain anti-inflammatory eicosanoid balance lowering pain, breast density, endometriosis risks associating to estrogen excess overlooked as solely a structural component.

Matching Multivitamin - As per follow up testing, a matching high quality 'nutrient insurance' multivitamin filling precise vitamin and mineral gaps rounded out by separate targeted doses of key inadequacies including magnesium, B-vitamins, zinc etc. helps sustain improvements initiated through the rebalancing phases correcting deficiency drivers.

Appropriately selected, high quality supplements prevent the tendency to revert back as reserves deplete with life's usual demands by providing consistent base support.

Strategic Detox Practices

While intensive detox practices need moderation for those currently recovering and regulating cycles due to potential adverse effects from sudden burdening of pathways, planned periodic cleansing provides immense value long term by reducing inflammatory and xenobiotic variables which tip the balance towards dysfunction over time.

Some strategic detoxes include:

Overnight Liver Flush - Periodic gentle 12 hour liver flushes via lemon juice, Epsom salt baths and milk thistle before bed safely enhance biliary drainage lowering reabsorption of estrogen metabolites and inflammatory mediators stalled in enterohepatic circulation promoting ongoing health of this vital organ.

Seasonal Cleanses - 7-14 day immune supporting cleanses tied to seasonal change using traditional alternatives like Triphala, Amalaki, Guduchi, Neem, Turmeric, Manjisthadi etc. reduce inflammatory and allergic undercurrents accumulated over months which indirectly worsen hormonal balance through crosstalk mechanisms. Guidance from an Ayurvedic practitioner ensures proper selection of cleansing herbs suiting your current health status.

Soothing Elimination Support - Natural aperients like slippery elm, marshmallow root, aloeVera etc. promote improved intestinal transit time and motility for weeks at a turn instead of stimulatory laxatives allowing gentle release of lodged estrogens and toxins without irritating conditions like leaky gut exacerbating issues.

Skin Brushing and Detox Baths - Using a natural fiber skin brush for lymphatic drainage weekly en-route to showering or adding bath salts, essential oils, Epsom salts, apple cider vinegar, bentonite clay etc. to your soak a few nights monthly enhances toxin removal through pores and ritual relaxation - easing pathways without drastic techniques.

The goal lies in providing your inner ecosystem a Spring cleaning consistently without sudden extreme protocols - easing accumulation gently through seasonal, monthly and weekly cleansing practices maintaining vibrancy.

Working with Your Doctor

While this guide aims to provide an extensively researched resource equipping you with tangible dietary, lifestyle, nutraceutical recommendations for improving estrogen metabolism towards balance guided by testing - working with a functional medicine practitioner or naturopath in person provides immense value through:

Ongoing Assessment

Symptoms, timeline, dietary inputs, supplements taken, lab markers, genetic SNPs etc form an elaborate matrix of insight across months. An experienced clinician pieces together connections and correlations to pinpoint very specific areas needing focus.

Troubleshooting Challenges

Plateaus, menstrual irregularities, weight loss resistance, low libido etc can arise despite interventions through complex drivers like adrenal imbalance, thyroid dysfunction or microbiome disruption that require expertise.

Medication and Testing Guidance

Navigating when to get off birth control, interpreting hormone, infection or allergy panels along with customized bioidentical hormones, adrenal adaptogens, testing beyond labs covered here etc requires skill.

Accountability and Validation

Having an authority you are accountable to weekly who tracks progress, provides troubleshooting, hand-holding support and most importantly validates efforts into better quality of life provides great mental relief motivating consistency.

While functional tests can be expensive, working step wise with a practitioner leveraging insurance covered labs allows maximizing benefits possible within your circumstances.

Certified ACN/CFM clinicians schooled in root cause resolution of complex hormonal cases through diet versus just medicating symptoms sets you up for genuine life-long healing success.

Troubleshooting Challenges

Despite your best efforts, intermittent back-tracking is part of recovery. Here are some key reasons and solutions:

Blood Sugar Imbalances

The post-detox phase often sees energy crashes, cravings for caffeine, chocolate etc as the body readjusts. Supporting stable blood sugar through adequate fiber, protein, healthy fats in meals while limiting refined carbohydrates and spacing meals prevents reactive eating.

Die-Off Symptoms

As pathogenic microbes linked to estrogen metabolism pathways die, they release endotoxins temporarily exacerbating fatigue, brain fog etc. Activated charcoal, electrolytes, glutathione foods and rest aid safe passage through adjustment reactions.

Stalled Weight Loss

Often rapid initial drops in inflammation provides weight release then plateaus as true metabolic healing kicks in. Further lower abdominal and hip area fat by emphasizing muscle building circulation, stress regulation, targeted high intensity workouts and patience trusting the process.

Lingering Digestive Issues Underlying infections, low pancreatic enzymes, bile acid insufficiencies, food sensitivities etc can continue until specifically treated hindering improvement through nutrient malabsorption, inflammation and indirectly hindering homeostasis through interconnected feedback loops.

Working back systematically from symptoms to root causes using lab testing for redirection is key. The wisdom lies in viewing lingering issues as helpful biological messengers drawing attention to areas needing modification for full healing.

Have faith in your body's potential supported by nutritional healing wisdom free of dogma or limitation.

Transitioning to Maintenance Phase

As intensive interventions taper down into integrated lifestyle habits and consciousness, sustaining improvement without burnout requires finding your version of what "living well" means day to day.

On the dietary nutrition front, having the foundations of real, whole foods, moderation of culprit substances, avoidance of sensitives, emphasis of protective categories ingrained as habits means you can enjoy the occasional dessert without remorse or drastic backslides.

Similarly, on the lifestyle realm, as keystone routines like working out become fun social activities, productive work outputs become automated, taking pause for mini-mediations becomes second nature, you move towards consistency which enhances vitality.

There will always be days of feasting, drinking or lost sleep. But resetting with veggie juices, calming teas, massage, sauna, nature walks, balances indulgence without militant extremes.

Trust in your body's wisdom. Each small choice adds up. Follow what makes you feel nourished. The rest unravels with time.

Conclusion

We've covered an extensive amount of evidence-based education around dysfunctional estrogen metabolism, steps to assess your hormone health, detailed dietary and lifestyle interventions in a pragmatic 28-day protocol with real life templates for meal planning, recipes and rhythm attunement alongside symptom alleviating nutritional supplementation.

You now possess a comprehensive understanding into the intricacies surrounding hormonal equilibrium and are equipped with tangible tools to reclaim balance through natural methods using food as medicine, liver supporting detox practices, stress busting techniques and targeted nutraceuticals.

While the specifics of this condition may seem complex on surface level dives, my hope is the simplified frameworks provided in this guide empowers you to become your own health advocate.

Hormones don't work in isolation but rather through an interconnected matrix with influence from the hypothalamus pituitary axis, thyroid health, adrenal function, blood sugar regulation, gut microbiome communication and much more.

Rest assured perfect lab numbers or lack of symptoms doesn't automatically equate complete healing. The human body is designed to handle temporary fluxes and emphasizes homeostasis through inbuilt buffering capacity.

But just like overdrawing on a bank account inevitably causes issues in the long run if spending outweighs earning and savings capacity, so do unaddressed stressors and dietary drivers which tip the scale towards dysfunction in the realm of hormones.

Through consciously engineered nutrition upgrading, stress resilience practices, appropriate testing, liver supporting detox regimes and an attitude of compassionate patience with ourselves and our healing journey - we can gradually guide our bodies back into alignment preventing long term issues of estrogen excess.

The intensive 28 day protocol detailed here provides a structured template easing guesswork while kickstarting change through high impact interventions across food, lifestyle and targeted supplementation in a step-wise pragmatic blueprint personalized to your unique needs.

But lasting success extends beyond just 4 weeks of effort no matter how Herculean. Integration of core principles learnt into daily living for months on end is where the transformation truly solidifies.

By internalizing key dietary guidelines of emphasizing hormone harmonizing foods, minimizing intake of disruptive compounds and ensuring adequate nutritional co-factors for optimal metabolism, you set yourself up for success in the long run.

Through layered deployment of proven stress busting practices, mindset shifts, movement routines and environmental upgrades tailored to your life minimizes the tendency of backslides and plateaus in progress so commonly witnessed.

There will invariably be ups and downs on the path as hormones wax and wane through menstrual cycles, seasons change, unforeseen circumstances arise and immunity fluctuates but do know that you are now infinitely better equipped to handle fluctuation.

Much like mastering culinary skills, musical instruments or any creative endeavor takes showing up day after day building slowly upon foundations learnt to translate knowledge into habit into mastery.

So too realizing lasting freedom from the uncomfortable symptoms of estrogen dominance requires consistency bridging moments into months through invariant core routines while adapting specifics to the day's needs.

But through celebrating small daily progress realised from mood improvements, better energy levels, reduced cravings to the bigger milestones of finally getting your period back, fitting into old jeans, sleeping well, the motivation for perseverance builds its own momentum expanding possibilities.

You CAN heal because your body WANTS to find homeostasis by design. Support it by consciously doing a little better each day listening to its whisper and it will respond with transformation beyond what you conceive possible at the moment!

The safe, layered, evidence based battle-tested recommendations within this guide converge into your personal roadmap custom fit for your unique history, priorities, possibilities and future growth.

Now grounded with education on what drives estrogen metabolism Awry, equipped with practical solutions across diet, nutrition, lifestyle, environment and mindset to course correct dysfunctional patterns plus armed with specific testing protocols to validate improvements in biomarkers along the way – you are ready!

The most challenging yet rewarding journeys often start with a single step. By reading this far seeking solutions for a better quality of life, you have already begun the first step shifting awake from suffering onto possibility.

Progress will ebb and peak in waves. But stay consistent corporating core methodologies day by day. Celebrate and course-correct. And witness your victorious emergence reclaiming harmonious balance from the inside out.

You've got this! Here's to Women reclaiming daily health, hormone equilibrium and living life fully on their own terms!

About the Author

As a doctor of naturopathic medicine and certified health coach, Dr. Omolola Habib is dedicated to guiding people on their personalized path to better wellbeing.

Dr. Habib's passion for holistic healing stems from her own health journey. After struggling with hormone issues for years, she found answers in integrative medicine. Now she wants to pay that help forward.

In her book "Balancing Hormones, Easing Symptoms," Dr. Habib simplifies the complex science behind hormonal balance into an actionable 28-day plan. With clarity and care, she helps readers pinpoint root causes and find relief from estrogen dominance symptoms.

Her integrative approach draws on years of specialized training along with intuition nurtured through deep listening of clients' needs. She believes optimal health manifests when we address the whole self — body, mind and spirit.